Acknowledgements

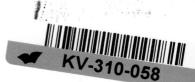

While writing this book I have received help from many people and I thank them sincerely.

Professor J. Vallance-Owen has been a source of encouragement and advice, and has kindly written the foreword.

Dr. D. R. Taylor gave generously of his time while reading my rough drafts and providing much helpful criticism. Dr. J. R. Hayes and Dr. H. Taggart gave advice in a number of areas. Others have helped with certain specific sections and these include Dr. B. Craig (Paediatrics), Dr. S. Creswell (Dermatology), Dr. J. Douglas (Renal Medicine), Dr. C. Humphries (Haematology), Dr. J. P. Jamison (Physiology), Dr. M. Lewis (Biochemistry), Dr J. K. McMullan (Endocrinology), Dr. J. D. Merrett (Statistics), Dr. K. Porter (Immunology) and Dr. N. Scott (Psychiatry). The questions have also been read and used by candidates preparing for M.R.C.P. Part I. Their comments and reactions have been especially valuable.

However, multiple choice questions inevitably generate some controversy and the final responsibility for the answers in this book is my own.

To my wife who put up with true and false answers at the breakfast table, more than thanks are due.

Multiple Choice Questions in Medicine

for the MRCP Examination (Part 1)

P. Bell MRCP
Registrar in General Medicine
Belfast City Hospital

with a Foreword by
J. Vallance-Owen

WRIGHT · PSG

Bristol   London   Boston
1981

Published by:
John Wright & Sons Ltd., 823–825 Bath Road, Bristol BS4 5NU, England
John Wright PSG Inc., 545 Great Road, Littleton, Massachusetts 01460, U.S.A.

First published, 1981
Reprinted, 1982

British Library Cataloguing in Publication Data
Bell, P.
    Multiple choice questions in medicine for the
    MRCP examination
    1. Medicine—Problems, exercises, etc.
    I. Title
    610.76   R834.5

ISBN 0 7236 0630 7

Library of Congress Catalog Card Number: 81–52682

Printed in Great Britain by
John Wright & Sons (Printing) Ltd at The Stonebridge Press, Bristol BS4 5NU

Contents

Foreword	vii
Introduction	ix
Anatomy	1
Biochemistry	5
Cardiology	9
Dermatology	19
Endocrinology and Metabolic Diseases	21
Gastroenterology	33
Genetics	43
Haematology	45
Immunology	55
Infectious and Tropical Diseases	59
Microbiology	69
Neurology	73
Occupational Diseases	83
Ophthalmology	85
Paediatrics	89
Pathology	99
Pharmacology	103
Physiology	113
Psychiatry	115
Poisoning	123
Renal Diseases	127
Respiratory Medicine	135
Rheumatology	145
Sexually Transmitted Diseases	153
Statistics	155
Symptoms and Signs	159

Foreword

by J. VALLANCE-OWEN
Professor of Medicine
The Queen's University of Belfast

Well constructed multiple choice questions are now recognised internationally as an efficient means for the assessment of knowledge, and are used for this purpose by many examining bodies. Although many people have a really excellent knowledge of medicine and its associated subjects, they often are not able to answer satisfactorily MCQ's and there is, undoubtedly, a technique for doing so.

The questions in this volume have been prepared primarily for use by those who are preparing for an examination such as MRCP (UK). They include not only questions relating to General (Internal) Medicine but also its various specialties and allied basic sciences, the latter having now become part of the re-constructed MRCP (UK). In the answering key there is not only the answer itself but often some further information about the point.

To use these questions to the best advantage is to do them on a strictly timed basis, for two of the greatest mistakes in answering MCQ's are either to run out of time i.e. to be left with ten questions to answer in three minutes, which is impossible, or to go too fast and have an hour left, having done the questions to the best of your ability. This latter situation is even worse than the former as, so often, your second thoughts, as you go through the questions again, are wrong.

I have encouraged Dr. Patrick Bell in this idea and he has produced a wide range of questions designed to test knowledge and skill in many aspects of medical practice and associated basic sciences. Anyone preparing for MRCP (UK) cannot familiarise themselves too much with the type of questions which are asked and which are put down in this book.

Introduction

This book is designed for those taking the first part of the examination for membership of the Royal College of Physicians. It may also be of use to Final MB and other postgraduate students.

MRCP Part 1 is a 2½-hour examination consisting of 60 multiple choice questions each with 5 parts. It covers in detail a wide range of topics in internal medicine and will increasingly test knowledge of basic sciences. To pass you must not only acquire sufficient knowledge, but also master the technique of doing multiple choice questions.

Acquiring the Knowledge
1. Plan your reading
Extensive reading is required, but remember that your time is limited. Your reading must be organised. Some candidates choose one of the large comprehensive textbooks of medicine and read it from cover to cover. Certainly most of the information is there, but it can be tedious. Others choose smaller monographs on the various topics. This is more interesting, but can mean using many different and expensive books.

Both these, as well as other, methods have been successfully used. Whatever method you decide upon, a little time spent planning your approach will be repaid.

2. Read widely
An examination consisting of sixty multiple choice questions can cover a wide range of subjects. Therefore you must read widely. Big subjects such as neurology and cardiology should be covered in depth. But other fringe subjects like tropical medicine and statistics also need some time spent on them. When all the questions from the fringe subjects are added together they form a significant percentage of the total paper.

3. Know the basics
There is a widespread belief that MRCP Part 1 concentrates on the small print. While multiple choice questions lend themselves to testing fine detail, the extent of this is overestimated in the case of MRCP. The rare disorders do come up, but the bulk of the questions are about common conditions. If one has time to read the small print it is better to know the rare manifestations of common conditions rather than the common manifestations of rare disorders.

While it is important to use modern text-books, the examination does not test up-to-the-minute research developments. Stick to established and currently held dogma. But do not get so lost in learning facts that you forget underlying principles. A little time on applied physiology will be well spent.

Mastering the Technique

1. The scoring system

Each question contains a single statement followed by five possible completions. Any, none, or all of the completed statements may be true. You can respond 'true', 'false' or 'don't know'. Each correct response receives one mark, and each incorrect response loses one mark. You receive a zero mark for each 'don't know'.

2. The marking system

You should study the instructions on marking the answer sheet issued by the colleges in their examination regulations.

The questions most people ask are 'What mark is needed to pass?', and 'On how many questions should I commit myself to a definite "true" or "false" when there is a risk of losing marks for wrong answers?'

No definite answer can be given to either question, but in general it is felt that a mark of above 60 per cent (or 180 out of 300) is needed to pass, remembering that the exact pass mark varies on each occasion that the examination takes place. There are two broad approaches used to achieve success.

The first approach is the cautious one and suggests that you mark 'true' or 'false' only those questions about which you are sure or nearly sure, and leave the rest as 'don't know'. Allowing for a few mistakes, if you commit yourself on about 210 parts, you would feel hopeful of passing, but remember you have virtually no chance if you answer less than 180 parts.

The more aggressive approach is based on the fact that guessing 'true' or 'false' gives a 50 per cent chance of being correct: an informed guess should have a better chance. Therefore it is claimed that by answering nearly all the questions, including those you are unsure about, you should do better than by being cautious. It is odd, though, how often informed guesses are incorrect!

Candidates have passed using either approach, and many probably fall between the two extremes. Much depends on your temperament. Try to work out which way is best for you while doing practice questions.

3. Practice

You must get practice with multiple choice questions. One selection is that released in book form by the colleges. All these questions have come up in previous papers and could come up again. Other questions available through correspondence courses vary in quality.

In doing practice questions you will see that certain subjects lend themselves to the multiple choice format. Try in your reading to focus on those pieces of information, which could be easily included.

4. Ambiguous questions

Candidates constantly complain that certain questions are ambiguous, and of course in badly set papers this can be true. There is nothing more annoying than knowing the details of a particular question, but being unable to answer because of confused wording. In general things are improving and the MRCP Part 1 questions are of a high standard. Genuine ambiguity is rare. Remember that a fairly obvious answer is usually required. You can get into trouble by thinking too deeply!

Using this Book

The questions in this book are designed to be like those that you will see in the examination. I hope they will be helpful in revising the basic knowledge required, and in practising and developing the answering technique.

You are best to do them under examination conditions. Set yourself a given number of questions in the appropriate space of time. Do not look at the answers until you have finished those questions.

The question format in this book is identical with that in the membership examination. The distribution of questions amongst the various subjects is roughly comparable. However, the colleges have indicated that there will be an increasing number of questions on the basic sciences. In the past there have usually been questions on anatomy, physiology, immunology and statistics. Biochemistry, microbiology and pathology are now to be covered. It is hard to assess in advance the range and difficulty of the questions in these new subjects. However, I have included some questions, which I hope will at least stimulate interest and relevant reading.

I hope the comments in the answer section will cope with some of the points that may arise. There is not enough space to deal with everything fully, but I would hope that certain points are highlighted which, though important, are not given much space in the textbooks.

It is important that you realise why you have gone wrong in a particular question. Was it carelessness, a definite lack of factual knowledge or ignorance of basic principles? If you can answer these questions and go on to correct the deficiency, then this book may be of some help.

Finally, if there are answers with which after consideration you still disagree, I would like to hear from you. Then I may learn something as well!

Anatomy

1. **Of nerves leaving the skull—**
   a. The optic nerve goes through the superior orbital fissure
   b. The mandibular nerve goes through the foramen ovale
   c. The glossopharyngeal nerve goes through the jugular foramen
   d. The 12th nerve goes through the foramen lacerum
   e. The 7th nerve goes through the foramen rotundum

2. **The median nerve supplies—**
   a. Brachioradialis
   b. Adductor pollicis
   c. Flexor carpi ulnaris
   d. Flexor pollicis brevis
   e. Palmar interossei

3. **The superior mesenteric artery—**
   a. Arises at the level of the fourth lumbar vertebra
   b. Lies behind the pancreas at its origin
   c. Passes above the third part of the duodenum
   d. Supplies large intestine as far as the sigmoid colon
   e. Supplies the liver

4. **Structures situated in the pons include the—**
   a. Fourth nerve nucleus
   b. Vestibular nuclei
   c. Nucleus ambiguus
   d. Reticular formation
   e. Olivary nucleus

Answers overleaf

1. a. False   It goes through the optic canal
   b. True
   c. True   Along with the jugular vein, the vagus nerve and the accessory nerve
   d. False   It goes through the hypoglossal canal
   e. False   It goes through the internal auditory meatus

2. a. False   It is supplied by the radial nerve
   b. False   It is supplied by the ulnar nerve
   c. False   This and part of flexor digitorum profundus are the only flexors of the forearm supplied by the ulnar nerve. The median supplies the others
   d. True   Flexor pollicis brevis, abductor pollicis brevis, opponens pollicis and the lateral two lumbricals are the only muscles of the hand supplied by the median nerve
   e. False

3. a. False   It arises at the level of the first lumbar vertebra
   b. True
   c. False   It passes below
   d. False   It supplies as far as the splenic flexure
   e. False   The liver is supplied by the right and left hepatic arteries, which are branches of the coeliac artery

4. a. False   It is in the midbrain
   b. True
   c. False   It is in the medulla
   d. True
   e. False   It is in the medulla

5. **In the foetal circulation—**
   a. The liver receives its blood supply from the ductus venosus
   b. Most of the blood from the superior vena cava goes through the atrial septal defect
   c. The head and heart receive better oxygenated blood than the lower parts of the body
   d. The superior vena cava is derived from the right common cardinal vein
   e. The ductus arteriosus usually joins the aorta just distal to the origin of the left subclavian artery

Answers overleaf

5.   a.   False   The ductus venosus bypasses the liver to bring placental blood to the heart

      b.   False   That from the inferior vena cava is directed through the septum to supply oxygenated blood to the left side of the heart

      c.   True   Blood going to the lower parts is mixed with poorly oxygenated blood from the ductus arteriosus

      d.   True

      e.   True

Biochemistry

1. **Galactose—**
   a. Has the same molecular weight as glucose
   b. Is directly converted to glucose by the enzyme galactose oxidase
   c. Is formed when lactose is hydrolysed
   d. From the diet is stored in the liver as galactose-1-phosphate
   e. In the urine gives a positive test with Clinitest tablets

2. **Glycogen—**
   a. Is composed of a mixture of different hexoses
   b. Is broken down and synthesised using the same enzymes
   c. In muscle can be broken down and released into the bloodstream as glucose in response to hypoglycaemia
   d. Breakdown is increased by glucagon
   e. Is abnormal in structure in von Gierke's disease

3. **The tricarboxylic acid cycle (Krebs cycle)—**
   a. Is regulated by the concentration of oxaloacetate
   b. Takes place within the mitochondria
   c. Produces relatively more energy than does glycolysis for the equivalent amount of substrate
   d. Produces lactic acid as an important byproduct
   e. Provides substrates for amino acid synthesis

4. **Substances that can be classified as steroids include—**
   a. Chenodeoxycholic acid
   b. Prolactin
   c. Glucocerebroside
   d. β-carotene
   e. Testosterone

Answers overleaf

1. a. True   The only difference is the configuration of the radicals about one of the carbon atoms, i.e. they are epimers
    b. False   Galactose first is converted to galactose-1-phosphate by galactokinase and then to glucose-1-phosphate by another enzyme
    c. True   Glucose is the other product formed
    d. False   It is converted to glucose-6-phosphate and can then be stored as glycogen. Galactose-1-phosphate builds up in galactosaemia and causes liver damage
    c. True   It is a reducing sugar

2. a. False   It is composed of glucose only
    b. False   Different enzymes are involved
    c. False   Muscles lack the enzyme glucose-6-phosphatase, which is necessary to liberate free glucose. The liver is primarily responsible for maintaining blood glucose homeostasis
    d. True
    e. False   Glucose-6-phosphatase is deficient in von Gierke's and liberation of free glucose is the problem. Glycogen structure is abnormal in some of the other glycogen storage diseases

3. a. True
    b. True   Whereas glycolysis takes place outside the mitochondria
    c. True   Breakdown to very simple molecules (carbon dioxide and water) causes a great release of energy
    d. False   This is a byproduct of glycolysis
    e. True   For example α-ketoglutarate and succinate

4. a. True   A bile salt
    b. False   A polypeptide
    c. False   Glucocerebroside is a combination of glucose with a ceramide
    d. False
    e. True

5. **Insulin—**

    a.   Is a glycoprotein

    b.   Has a half-life in the circulation of 4 hours after intravenous injection

    c.   Increases protein synthesis from amino acids in muscle

    d.   Increases glucose uptake by the brain

    e.   Increases the activity of glycogen phosphorylase

Answers overleaf

5. a. False   It is a polypeptide
    b. False   It is less than 20 minutes
    c. True
    d. False   Insulin causes glucose uptake in muscle and adipose tissue
    e. False   Insulin increases the activity of the enzymes of glycogen synthesis

Cardiology

1. **Atrial myxoma—**
   a. Is the commonest primary tumour found in the heart
   b. Usually arises in the right atrium
   c. May be diagnosed by echocardiography
   d. May mimic mitral stenosis
   e. Is associated with constitutional symptoms

2. **Central cyanosis—**
   a. Is usually present where arterial P_{O_2} is less than 50 mmHg (6·7 kPa)
   b. Is present if the hands are blue and warm
   c. In those with right-to-left shunts can be completely corrected by inhalation of 100% oxygen
   d. Is seen in normal people at altitudes of 5000 feet
   e. Can be associated with hereditary haemorrhagic telangiectasia

3. **In the jugular venous pulse—**
   a. The level normally falls on inspiration
   b. The 'a' wave is due to atrial contraction
   c. The 'x' descent is due to blood entering the ventricles
   d. The 'v' wave is due to ventricular contraction
   e. The 'y' descent is reduced in tricuspid stenosis

4. **A fourth heart sound—**
   a. Is usually physiological, when heard in those under 30 years old
   b. Corresponds in timing to the 'a' wave of the jugular venous pulse
   c. May be an early sign of heart disease
   d. Is associated with a reduction in ventricular compliance
   e. Is a recognised feature of systemic hypertension

Answers overleaf

1. a. True
    b. False Usually in the left
    c. True But angiography may also be required
    d. True Dyspnoea, mid-diastolic murmurs, atrial fibrillation and systemic emboli all occur
    e. True But not always

2. a. True
    b. True Peripheral cyanosis without central cyanosis implies cold blue peripheries due to a poor circulation. If the circulation is good (i.e. the peripheries warm) and the hands are blue, central cyanosis must also be present
    c. False Remember that in right-to-left shunts blood is by-passing the lungs and no amount of inspired oxygen can completely make up for this
    d. False Higher altitudes of around 15,000 feet are required
    e. True Pulmonary arteriovenous fistulas are found and these cause right-to-left shunting

3. a. True Due to the lower intrathoracic pressure. In pericardial effusion the venous pressure increases on inspiration (Kussmaul's sign)
    b. True
    c. False It is due to atrial relaxation and/or the downward movement of the tricuspid valve ring with the onset of ventricular systole
    d. False It is due to venous filling of the atria
    e. True The 'y' descent is due to blood filling the right ventricle from the right atrium. This filling is reduced in tricuspid stenosis

4. a. False An audible fourth heart sound is always pathological
    b. True Both coincide with atrial contraction
    c. True Generally this is so while a third sound is generally a late sign. This is the sort of vague question which it can be wise not to answer!
    d. True Since the atrium must contract against greater ventricular resistance
    e. True Since the ventricular compliance is increased

5. **The intensity of a murmur—**
   a. From the right side of the heart is increased by expiration
   b. Of aortic stenosis is increased by amyl nitrite
   c. Of hypertrophic obstructive cardiomyopathy is increased by Valsalva manoeuvre
   d. Of mitral stenosis is proportional to severity
   e. Of aortic incompetence is increased by hand-grip exercise

6. **Prominent pulmonary arteries on chest X-ray may be seen in—**
   a. Ventricular septal defect
   b. Valvular pulmonary stenosis
   c. Fallot's tetralogy
   d. Severe mitral stenosis
   e. Multiple pulmonary emboli

7. **Constrictive pericarditis—**
   a. Characteristically produces acute pulmonary oedema
   b. Follows rheumatic fever
   c. Characteristically causes gross cardiomegaly on chest X-ray
   d. May be caused by rheumatoid arthritis
   e. Causes increased cardiac pulsation on fluoroscopy

8. **Cardiac output is increased by—**
   a. Increased β-sympathetic nervous system activity
   b. Administration of digoxin to normal subjects at rest
   c. Increasing heart rate in response to exercise
   d. Increasing ventricular end-diastolic volume
   e. Increasing ventricular after-load

Answers overleaf

5. a. False   Inspiration decreases intrathoracic pressure and causes blood to enter the right side of the heart
   b. True   Amyl nitrite lowers peripheral resistance and increases the gradient between the left ventricle and aorta
   c. True   The heart is made smaller and obstruction increased
   d. False   The length of the murmur is proportional to severity
   e. True   Hand-grip exercise increases peripheral resistance and therefore increases the gradient between the aorta and left ventricle in diastole

6. a. True   Due to increased blood flow
   b. True   Due to post-stenotic dilatation
   c. False   The outflow obstruction is subvalvular and there is no post-stenotic dilatation. Blood flow through the pulmonary arteries is much reduced
   d. True   Due to pulmonary hypertension
   e. True   Again due to pulmonary hypertension

7. a. False
   b. False   Virtually never happens
   c. False   The constricted heart is often of normal size
   d. True   With the decline of tuberculosis, this is now quite a common cause
   e. False   The ventricular movement is reduced

8. a. True   Heart rate and cardiac contraction are both increased
   b. False   In normal persons other compensatory mechanisms maintain the cardiac output at normal
   c. True   Obviously
   d. True   Starling's law
   e. False   The heart cannot work so well against increased resistance

9. **Ventricular aneurysms—**
    a. Are usually caused by rheumatic fever
    b. Cause recurrent ventricular tachycardia
    c. Are characteristically associated with persistent ST depression
    d. Cause cardiac failure
    e. Give rise to systemic emboli

10. **The ECG in acute pulmonary embolism characteristically shows—**
    a. Sinus bradycardia
    b. ST and T wave changes in V5 and V6
    c. Left axis shift
    d. Changes which may disappear in a few days
    e. Right bundle branch block

11. **Acute rheumatic fever—**
    a. Does not recur
    b. Follows streptococcal skin infections
    c. Is caused only by β-haemolytic streptococci of certain Griffith types
    d. Complicated by chorea rarely gives cardiac sequelae
    e. There may be a short P–R interval on ECG

12. **In pure mitral stenosis—**
    a. A third heart sound is heard
    b. The apex beat is displaced
    c. Infective endocarditis is a characteristic complication
    d. Women are affected more often than men
    e. A history of rheumatic fever is obtained in 95% of cases

13. **In mitral valve prolapse (floppy mitral valve syndrome)—**
    a. Chest pain may be the presenting symptom
    b. An opening snap may be heard
    c. The ECG may show inferolateral changes
    d. Echocardiography is useful diagnostically
    e. Endocarditis is a recognised complication

Answers overleaf

9. a. False
b. True This may cease after surgical correction
c. False ST elevation is characteristic
d. True
e. True

10. a. False Sinus tachycardia is usual. Chest pain and sinus bradycardia suggest an inferior myocardial infarction
b. False These changes are usually seen in the right ventricular
leads
c. False Right axis shift is usual
d. True
e. True

11. a. False
b. False It only occurs after throat infections
c. False Most of the Lancefield group A streptococci cause it
d. False Chorea often has cardiac sequelae
e. False It is long

12. a. False A third heart sound is due to ventricular filling and
this is impaired in mitral stenosis
b. False Unless mitral incompetence is present
c. False Incompetent valves are more often the seat of
endocarditis
d. True
e. False Percentage figures rarely appear unless they are clearly
incorrect. The figure here is much lower

13. a. True Mitral valve prolapse is popular in cardiological
circles and a question could just come up
b. False It is a mid-systolic click
c. True
d. True The posterior mitral valve leaflet is seen to open during
systole
e. True

14. **The first heart sound is loud in—**
    a. First degree heart block
    b. Wolff—Parkinson—White syndrome
    c. Mitral stenosis with a heavily calcified valve
    d. Aortic stenosis
    e. Hypertrophic obstructive cardiomyopathy

15. **Characteristic features of severe aortic stenosis are—**
    a. Exertional syncope
    b. Loud aortic second sound
    c. Blood pressure of 180/120 mmHg
    d. Left ventricular hypertrophy on ECG
    e. Catheter gradient of 60 mmHg across the valve

16. **In hypertrophic obstructive cardiomyopathy—**
    a. Mitral incompetence may develop
    b. Use of digoxin is important in the early stages
    c. A family history is nearly always obtained
    d. Pregnancy is well tolerated
    e. Syncope is a characteristic symptom

17. **Characteristic features of Eisenmenger's syndrome complicating atrial septal defect include—**
    a. Development before 20 years of age
    b. Giant 'a' waves
    c. Pulmonary incompetence
    d. Differential cyanosis
    e. Necessity of surgical correction

Answers overleaf

14. a. False The P–R interval is long and the first heart sound varies inversely in intensity with the length of the P–R interval
 b. True The P–R interval is short
 c. False The heavily calcified valve cannot close rapidly enough to produce the classic loud first heart sound
 d. False There is no connection
 e. False

15. a. True The cardiac output cannot increase in response to the increased demand during exercise
 b. False The aortic second sound should be soft
 c. False A low pulse pressure would be expected
 d. True
 e. True

16. a. True This probably results from distortion of the mitral valve by the hypertrophic left ventricle
 b. False Digoxin makes the heart smaller and may increase obstruction
 c. False This occurs in about 30% of cases
 d. True A little surprising
 e. True

17. a. False It usually occurs in later life
 b. True Due to pulmonary hypertension
 c. True Again due to pulmonary hypertension
 d. False Differential cyanosis (i.e. cyanosis of the lower part of the body more than the upper part of the body) is seen in Eisenmenger's syndrome complicating patent ductus
 e. False If the septal defect is closed an intolerable burden is placed on the right side of the heart

18. **A prolonged Q–T interval on ECG may be seen with—**
    a. Hypercalcaemia
    b. Digitalis therapy
    c. Ischaemic heart disease
    d. Hypothermia
    e. Quinidine therapy

19. **In left ventricular failure the following parameters are increased—**
    a. Pulmonary venous pressure
    b. Left ventricular end-diastolic pressure
    c. Lung compliance
    d. Po_2
    e. Pco_2

20. **The first heart sound is variable in intensity in—**
    a. Complete heart block
    b. Ventricular tachycardia
    c. Right bundle branch block
    d. Wolff–Parkinson–White syndrome
    e. Atrial fibrillation

Answers overleaf

18.   a.   False   The Q–T interval in short
      b.   False   Again here the Q–T interval is reduced
      c.   True
      d.   True
      e.   True

19.   a.   True
      b.   True
      c.   False   The oedematous lungs are harder to move
      d.   False   The P_{O_2} is reduced
      e.   False   Hyperventilation allows P_{CO_2} to be excreted since it diffuses more easily across the alveolar membrane

20.   a.   True   The intensity of the first heart sound is proportional to the position of the valve cusps at the beginning of systole. In complete heart block ventricular systole occurs at quite irregular times in relation to the position of the valve cusps
      b.   True   As in complete heart block atrial and ventricular contraction is dissociated
      c.   False   Slightly increased splitting may be detectable
      d.   False   The first heart sound is consistently loud
      e.   True

Dermatology

1. **Itch is characteristic of—**
   a. Secondary syphilis
   b. Dermatitis herpetiformis
   c. Atopic eczema
   d. Scabies
   e. Psoriasis

2. **Involvement of the skin of the hands is characteristic of—**
   a. Herpes zoster
   b. Pompholyx
   c. Anthrax
   d. Pityriasis rosea
   e. Acne vulgaris

3. **Characteristic features of pemphigus vulgaris include—**
   a. Highest incidence in old age
   b. Subepidermal bullae
   c. Mucosal involvement
   d. Intense itch
   e. Presence of auto-antibody in skin

4. **The Koebner phenomenon is a recognised feature of—**
   a. Dermatitis herpetiformis
   b. Psoriasis
   c. Acne vulgaris
   d. Lichen planus
   e. Molluscum contagiosum

5. **Pitting of the finger nails is seen in—**
   a. Dermatitis herpetiformis
   b. Psoriasis
   c. Alopecia areata
   d. Acne rosacea
   e. Arsenic poisoning

Answers overleaf

1. a. False Virtually never
   b. True Itch is often so intense that bullae do not survive intact, and excoriation predominates
   c. True
   d. True
   e. False Psoriasis is occasionally itchy but not typically so

2. a. False The face or trunk is usually involved
   b. True Palms and soles are usually affected
   c. True Contact is often via the hands
   d. False The trunk is mainly involved
   e. False Areas with plenty of sebaceous glands, like the face and trunk are involved

3. a. False It is a disease of middle age
   b. False They are intra-epidermal. In dermatitis herpetiformis and pemphigoid they are sub-epidermal
   c. True Mucosal involvement is rare in dermatitis herpetiformis and pemphigoid
   d. False Again unlike dermatitis herpetiformis
   e. True This can be demonstrated by immunofluorescence. Serum antibodies are also present

4. a. False The Koebner phenomenon is the induction at the site of trauma of skin changes present elsewhere
   b. True It is particularly characteristic of psoriasis
   c. False
   d. True
   e. True A rare cause

5. a. False
   b. True
   c. True
   d. False
   e. False But horizontal white lines are found on the nails (Mees' lines)

Endocrinology and Metabolic Diseases

1. **Recognised features of acromegaly include —**
   a. Hypertension
   b. Dry skin
   c. Goitre
   d. Hypophosphataemia
   e. Glucose intolerance

2. **In a 60-year-old lady suspected of having panhypopituitarism features that would be characteristic of this diagnosis include —**
   a. Pale skin and a haemoglobin of 6·0 g/dl (6·0 g/100 ml)
   b. History of failure to lactate after last child
   c. Potassium of 2·0 mmol/l
   d. Absent body hair
   e. Obesity

3. **Drugs that cause goitre include —**
   a. Neo-mercazole (Carbimazole)
   b. Digoxin
   c. Lithium
   d. Iodine
   e. Streptomycin

4. **A newly diagnosed 16-year-old diabetic boy —**
   a. Should receive a reduced calorie intake for his age
   b. Should have all urine tests showing blue before discharge
   c. Should be allowed to continue playing rugby
   d. Should be tried on a biguanide before resorting to insulin
   e. Will have, in response to a glucose load, insulin levels about 50% of normal

Answers overleaf

1. a. True
   b. False Excess sweating is characteristic
   c. True The thyroid is not spared from the general viscero-megaly
   d. False Hyperphosphataemia is seen occasionally
   e. True

2. a. False Pallor without anaemia is characteristic of hypo-pituitarism. If anaemia occurs it is mild
   b. True This would suggest post-partum haemorrhage leading to pituitary necrosis as the cause
   c. False
   d. True
   e. False They are usually asthenic

3. a. True Most goitrogens block thyroid hormone synthesis. The gland hypertrophies to maintain the euthyroid state. This is said to be mediated by TSH, but is in fact elevated only occasionally
   b. False
   c. True Other goitrogens include phenylbutazone, PAS, resorcinol and some vegetables
   d. True
   e. False

4. a. False He needs normal amounts of calories to grow, but refined carbohydrate is restricted
   b. False Although tight sugar control is now the aim, his sugars are likely to fall when he resumes school and games. In any case some young diabetics find that reduction in insulin dose over the first few months is necessary (honeymoon period)
   c. True He may need to alter his insulin dose, or take extra sugar before a match
   d. False Very few young diabetics do not need insulin
   e. False They are much lower

5. **Hypoglycaemia is a recognised feature of—**
    a. von Gierke's disease
    b. Renal glycosuria
    c. Acute alcoholic intoxication
    d. Phenylketonuria
    e. Primary hepatoma

6. **Recognised features of Hashimoto's disease include—**
    a. High titre of thyroid autoantibodies
    b. Exophthalmos
    c. Hypothyroidism
    d. Presence of parietal cell antibodies
    e. Enlargement of the goitre when 1-thyroxine is given

7. **Recognised features of thyrotoxicosis include—**
    a. Deafness
    b. Pretibial myxoedema
    c. Ataxic gait
    d. Glycosuria
    e. Unilateral exophthalmos

8. **Investigation of a case of hypothyroidism due to primary involvement of the thyroid gland may show—**
    a. No rise in TSH in response to intravenous TRH
    b. An abnormally low ESR
    c. Reduced thyroid binding globulin
    d. Increased creatinine phosphokinase
    e. Delta waves on ECG

9. **In Paget's disease—**
    a. Men are more often affected than women
    b. Bones are stronger than normal
    c. Optic atrophy may occur
    d. High output cardiac failure is a common cause of death
    e. Urinary hydroxyproline excretion is increased

Answers overleaf

5. a. True   Glucose-6-phosphatase is deficient
    b. False Losses are small
    c. True   Beware of correction without giving vitamin supplements, as Wernicke's encephalopathy can be precipitated
    d. False
    e. True

6. a. True
    b. True   Although of course it is commoner in thyrotoxicosis
    c. True
    d. True   Association with other organ specific autoimmune diseases is common
    e. False Thyroxine often causes the goitre to regress

7. a. False A feature of hypothyroidism
    b. True   And is especially associated with exophthalmos and a high level of long-acting thyroid stimulator (LATS)
    c. False Ataxia is occasionally seen in myxoedema
    d. True
    e. True   Although retro-orbital tumours need to be considered

8. a. False The hypothalamo-pituitary axis is responsive to TRH and high TSH levels are produced, unlike hyperthyroidism and hypopituitarism
    b. False It is moderately elevated
    c. False
    d. True   A myopathy is seen occasionally, while a raised CPK is quite common
    e. False These are seen in Wolff–Parkinson–White syndrome

9. a. True
    b. False Although bones may be thickened they are weaker than usual. Pathological fractures are a complication
    c. True   It is a rare complication
    d. False It is quite rare
    e. True   As in other disorders where bone breakdown allows hydroxyproline release from collagen matrix

10. Causes of hypercalcaemia include—

    a. Hypomagnesaemia
    b. Sarcoidosis
    c. Osteoporosis
    d. Thyrotoxicosis
    e. Frusemide

11. Osteoporosis—

    a. Causes Looser's zones
    b. May complicate thyrotoxicosis
    c. Is associated with a raised alkaline phosphatase
    d. May result from long-term use of heparin
    e. Characteristically produces continuous bone pain

12. Causes of hypocalcaemia include—

    a. Acute pancreatitis
    b. Chronic pyelonephritis
    c. Hysterical overbreathing
    d. Cushing's syndrome
    e. Pseudo hypoparathyroidism

13. Hypercholesterolaemia—

    a. Is usually caused by deficiency of the enzyme lipoprotein lipase
    b. May present with arthritis
    c. Of severe degree is inherited as a dominant trait
    d. Is reversed by administration of bile salts
    e. Is a characteristic feature of primary biliary cirrhosis

Answers overleaf

10. a. False
    b. True   The mechanism is thought to be increased vitamin D sensitivity
    c. False   Remember that calcium, phosphate and alkaline phosphatase are all normal
    d. True   It is a rare complication
    e. False   The thiazide diuretics cause hypercalcaemia, but the loop diuretics cause increased calcium excretion

11. a. False   They are found in osteomalacia
    b. True
    c. False
    d. True   Though this is not a very common situation
    e. False   The pain is typically intermittent associated with fractures, which then heal up. Osteomalacia produces continuous pain

12. a. True
    b. True   As with other causes of chronic renal failure
    c. False   This causes alkalosis and hence tetany by lowering the ionised calcium, but the total calcium (ionised and protein bound) is unaltered and this is what is usually measured
    d. False   Hypercalciuria is occasionally seen
    e. True   By end-organ insensitivity to parathormone

13. a. False   Lipoprotein lipase deficiency is responsible for hyper-chylomicronaemia, which is rare
    b. True
    c. True
    d. False   Cholestyramine which binds cholesterol containing bile salts is used
    e. True

14. **Recognised features of hyperparathyroidism include—**
    a. Normal alkaline phosphatase
    b. Reduction in hypercalcaemia after hydrocortisone
    c. Hyperphosphaturia
    d. Increased blood urea
    e. Increased urinary hydroxyproline

15. **Causes of increased bone density on X-ray include—**
    a. Hand—Schüller—Christian disease
    b. Prostatic secondaries
    c. Multiple myeloma
    d. Paget's disease
    e. Osteoporosis

16. **Features of Cushing's syndrome due to ectopic ACTH production which also help to differentiate from Cushing's syndrome due to a basophil adenoma include—**
    a. Skin pigmentation
    b. Marked hypokalaemia
    c. Suppression of cortisol after 2 mg dexamethasone 6-hourly for 2 days
    d. Males more commonly affected
    e. Grossly elevated ACTH levels

17. **Characteristic features of carcinoma of the thyroid include—**
    a. History of treatment of hyperthyroidism with radioactive iodine
    b. Increased uptake of iodine in the cancerous area as shown by a thyroid scan
    c. Hypocalcaemia in the medullary type
    d. Normal serum thyroxine
    e. Benefit from thyroxine in papillary type

Answers overleaf

14. a. True   The raised alkaline phosphatase reflects bone disease which is not always present
     b. False   This is the basis of a diagnostic test, since most other causes of hypercalcaemia will respond
     c. True   Parathormone increases phosphate excretion
     d. True   Renal failure may occur due to nephrocalcinosis
     e. True

15. a. False   Lytic lesions are characteristic
     b. True   With breast cancer, are the commonest causes of sclerotic secondaries
     c. False   'Punched-out' lesions are classic. More generalised bone thinning is also seen
     d. True
     e. False

16. a. False   It occurs in both
     b. True   In most cases of Cushing's syndrome hypokalaemia is mild but it can be severe in ectopic ACTH production
     c. False   Ectopic ACTH production does not suppress in the high dose dexamethasone suppression test, while cortisol production is suppressed in Cushing's due to a basophil adenoma
     d. True   Related to the higher incidence of oat cell carcinoma in males
     e. True   ACTH is much less markedly elevated in a basophil adenoma

17. a. False   No such association is proved
     b. False   Hot nodules are nearly always benign
     c. False   Although calcitonin tends to lower calcium, hypocalcaemia is rarely seen
     d. True
     e. True   Thyroxine is of less benefit in the other types

18. **In phaeochromocytoma—**
    a. Treatment of choice for an acute hypertensive episode is intravenous β-blockade
    b. An aura may precede the attack
    c. Paroxysmal hypotension is recognised
    d. There is an excess of 5-hydroxyindole acetic acid in the urine
    e. A family history of the disease may be obtained

19. **Pituitary diabetes insipidus is improved by—**
    a. Water restriction
    b. Glucagon
    c. Lithium
    d. Chlorpropamide
    e. Chlorthiazide

20. **Recognised features of Conn's syndrome include—**
    a. Low urinary potassium
    b. Tetany
    c. High renin levels
    d. Reduced sweat levels of sodium
    e. Polyuria

21. **In excessive antidiuretic hormone secretion—**
    a. Restriction of fluid intake may alleviate symptoms
    b. A history of head injury may be obtained
    c. Plasma osmolarity is increased
    d. Urinary sodium is low
    e. Ankle oedema is characteristic

22. **Glycosuria is a recognised finding in—**
    a. Acute intermittent porphyria
    b. Wilson's disease
    c. Hypothyroidism
    d. Galactosaemia
    e. Sub-arachnoid haemorrhage

Answers overleaf

18. a. False   A β-blocker alone allows uncontrolled α effects
     b. True
     c. True   Probably in those cases where adrenaline, with its vasodilator effects, is in excess
     d. False   It is adrenaline, noradrenaline and their derivatives that are found
     e. True   As may a history in the patient or his family of neurofibromatosis and medullary carcinoma of the thyroid

19. a. False   Water restriction and the failure of urine to concentrate is diagnostic but not therapeutic
     b. False
     c. False   Lithium causes diabetes insipidus
     d. True   Hypoglycaemia is a troublesome complication
     e. True   Is also useful in nephrogenic diabetes insipidus

20. a. False
     b. True   Due to alkalosis
     c. False   They are low
     d. True   As with urine
     e. True   ⁻Due to hypokalaemia

21. a. True   The problem is failure to excrete water, with resultant water overload
     b. True   Various intracranial disorders, e.g. trauma, infection and neoplasm, are among the many causes of this syndrome
     c. False   Haemodilution occurs
     d. False   Sodium excretion is not fundamentally affected
     e. False   Despite the water overload oedema is unusual

22. a. False
     b. True   Due to a renal tubular defect
     c. False
     d. False   Reducing sugar as galactose is detected in the urine, but not glucose
     e. True

23. **Hyperprolactinaemia is a recognised finding in —**
    a. Chlorpromazine therapy
    b. Breast cancer
    c. Hypothyroidism
    d. L-dopa therapy
    e. Chromophobe adenoma

24. **Causes of hirsutism include —**
    a. Addison's disease
    b. Adrenal carcinoma
    c. Thyrotoxicosis
    d. Phenytoin
    e. Polycystic ovary syndrome

25. **Causes of low urinary calcium include —**
    a. Renal tubular acidosis
    b. Cushing's syndrome
    c. Chronic glomerulonephritis
    d. Osteomalacia
    e. Paget's disease

Answers overleaf

23. a. True Chlorpromazine is a dopamine antagonist
    b. False There is no known association
    c. True
    d. False
    e. True These so-called 'non-secretory tumours' are the usual
           finding when a pituitary cause is present

24. a. False
    b. True And also causes Cushing's syndrome
    c. False But it does occasionally cause gynaecomastia
    d. True A reason for avoiding its use in adolescent females
    e. True

25. a. False Hypercalciuria is usual. Calculi may be seen
    b. False Hypercalciuria is occasionally seen
    c. True
    d. True
    e. False Hypercalciuria may be seen

Gastroenterology

1. A diagnosis of chronic active as against chronic persistent hepatitis is suggested by —
   a. Positive hepatitis B surface antigen
   b. Presence of renal tubular acidosis
   c. Positive antinuclear factor
   d. Liver biopsy showing mononuclear infiltration around the portal zones
   e. Two times elevation of the transaminases

2. Characteristic features of achalasia of the oesophagus include —
   a. Presentation before the age of 20
   b. Risk of post-cricoid carcinoma
   c. Failure of passage of endoscope into stomach
   d. Recurrent chest infections
   e. Narrowed corkscrew oesophagus on barium meal

3. Lower oesophageal sphincter tone is increased by —
   a. Stopping smoking
   b. Alkalis
   c. Metoclopramide
   d. Anticholinergics
   e. Truncal vagotomy

4. Complications more often associated with Crohn's disease than ulcerative colitis include —
   a. Sclerosing cholangitis
   b. Toxic megacolon
   c. Cholelithiasis
   d. Pyoderma gangrenosum
   e. Anal fistula

5. In the management of ulcerative colitis —
   a. Sulphasalazine is reserved for the acute exacerbation
   b. Colectomy generally leaves systemic complications unaltered
   c. Steroids prevent relapse
   d. Pregnancy is best avoided
   e. Regular B_{12} supplements are needed

Answers overleaf

1.   a.   False   It is associated with both types
      b.   True   There is a long list of other recognised associations with chronic active
      c.   True   In the 'lupoid' type
      d.   False   Quite in keeping with chronic persistent. In chronic active extension beyond the portal triad with piece-meal necrosis is characteristic
      e.   False   Occurs in both types

2.   a.   False   Presentation in the third and fourth decade is usual
      b.   False   Carcinoma is a complication, but post-cricoid carcinoma is particularly associated with iron deficiency
      c.   False   It passes easily
      d.   True
      e.   False   The upper oesophagus becomes widely dilated

3.   a.   True
      b.   False   Although they do provide symptomatic relief
      c.   True
      d.   False
      e.   False

4.   a.   False   Most of the liver complications are more common in ulcerative colitis
      b.   False
      c.   True   Due to failure of bile salt reabsorption
      d.   False
      e.   True

5.   a.   False   It is useful in preventing relapse as well
      b.   False   Liver, eye, skin and joint complications may all be helped. Note that sacro-iliitis generally is not helped
      c.   False
      d.   False   It is usually well tolerated
      e.   False B_{12} is absorbed normally, unlike Crohn's

6. **Aetiological factors in acute pancreatitis include—**
   a. Addison's disease
   b. Hyperparathyroidism
   c. Hypothermia
   d. Pancreatic carcinoma
   e. Hyperlipidaemia

7. **A patient has longstanding liver cirrhosis. Factors that suggest the possibility of liver cell carcinoma include—**
   a. Splenomegaly
   b. Development of an arterial bruit over the liver
   c. High titre of anti-mitochondrial antibody
   d. A sudden increase in the alkaline phosphatase level
   e. Ascites with a protein content of 40 g/l (4·0 g/100 ml)

8. **The C^{14} labelled bile salt breathalyser is characteristically abnormally elevated in patients with—**
   a. Ileal resection for Crohn's disease
   b. Coeliac disease
   c. Cystic fibrosis
   d. Jejunal diverticuli
   e. Biliary cirrhosis

9. **Malabsorption of pancreatic origin is characterised by—**
   a. Iron deficiency anaemia
   b. High faecal fat content
   c. High urinary indicans
   d. Less than 20% excretion in the urine of an oral load of D-xylose
   e. Low serum B_{12}

Answers overleaf

6. a. False
   b. True
   c. True
   d. True   Acute pancreatitis in the elderly should raise this possibility
   e. True   Particularly Fredrickson types I and V

7. a. False
   b. True   An arterial bruit usually indicates hepatoma or acute alcoholic hepatitis
   c. False   This is a feature of primary biliary cirrhosis
   d. True   Due to tumour obstructing the biliary tree
   e. True   Complicating.peritonitis would also give an exudate

8. a. True   Normally the C^{14} labelled bile salts are absorbed in the terminal ileum and recirculated. In terminal ileal disease the bile salts pass to the large intestine, where they are degraded, absorbed and then C^{14} is excreted in the lungs as carbon dioxide
   b. False
   c. False
   d. True   In blind loop syndromes bile salts are broken down
   e. False

9. a. False   Iron is absorbed in the acid environment of the duodenum as usual
   b. True   The grossest degrees of steatorrhoea are seen in pancreatic malabsorption
   c. False
   d. False   D-xylose absorption is abnormal in disorders affecting the intestinal mucosa
   e. False B_{12} absorption in the terminal ileum is not affected

10. **Characteristic features of an attack of ischaemic colitis include—**

   a. Inflamed mucosa on sigmoidoscopy
   b. Normal barium enema
   c. Necessity of emergency surgery
   d. Pyrexia
   e. Bloody diarrhoea

11. **Recognised features of coeliac disease include—**

   a. Mouth ulcers
   b. Presentation some months after gastrectomy
   c. Anterior uveitis
   d. Psoriasiform skin rash
   e. Family history of the disease

12. **Recognised features of large intestinal diverticular disease include—**

   a. Ascending colon as the most common site
   b. Malabsorption
   c. Massive bleeding
   d. Liver abscess
   e. Fistula formation

13. **In haemochromatosis—**

   a. Hepatoma complicates more often than in other forms of cirrhosis
   b. Chondro-calcinosis is a recognised feature
   c. Total iron binding capacity is elevated
   d. Desferrioxamine is the treatment of choice
   e. Cardiac failure is the main cause of death in untreated cases

14. **There is a recognised association between duodenal ulceration and—**

   a. Intracranial injury
   b. Pernicious anaemia
   c. Renal dialysis patients
   d. Gastric cancer
   e. Hepatic cirrhosis

Answers overleaf

10. a. False The problem is higher up at the splenic flexure
    b. False The 'thumbprint' sign due to mucosal oedema is characteristic
    c. False Conservative management is usually adequate
    d. True
    e. True

11. a. True
    b. True A subclinical defect may be exposed
    c. False
    d. False
    e. True

12. a. False Sigmoid colon is the commonest
    b. False Unlike jejunal diverticuli
    c. True
    d. True Due to portal pyaemia
    e. True

13. a. True A significant cause of death in treated cases
    b. True
    c. False Iron binding is saturated
    d. False Venesection is a quicker way of removing iron
    e. True Liver complications such as encephalopathy and oesophageal varices are less common than in other types of cirrhosis

14. a. True So-called 'Cushing's ulcer' may occur in the duodenum as well as the stomach
    b. False Hypochlorhydria prevails
    c. True Gastrin excretion may be impaired
    d. False
    e. True

15. **In severe pyloric stenosis findings include—**
    a. Hypokalaemia
    b. Raised urea
    c. Low urinary pH
    d. Hypochloraemia
    e. Tetany

16. **Characteristic features of Zollinger—Ellison syndrome include—**
    a. Diarrhoea
    b. Grossly exaggerated gastric acid response to intravenous pentagastrin
    c. Good results from tumour removal by partial pancreatectomy
    d. Death due to metastatic disease
    e. Association with other endocrine tumours

17. **In a patient with liver cirrhosis factors pointing towards an alcoholic aetiology include—**
    a. Peripheral neuropathy
    b. Splenomegaly
    c. Parotid enlargement
    d. Macronodular cirrhosis
    e. Hepatitis B surface antigen

18. **Characteristic features of the Budd—Chiari syndrome of hepatic vein obstruction include—**
    a. Association with polycythaemia vera
    b. Giant 'v' waves in the jugular venous pulse
    c. Patchy uptake of isotope in hepatic scintiscan
    d. Ascites
    e. Liver biopsy showing cirrhosis

Answers overleaf

15. a. True
     b. True
     c. True   Despite systemic alkalosis, the sodium-retaining mechanisms at the distal tubule take precedence and, with potassium already low, hydrogen ions are excreted in exchange for sodium
     d. True
     e. True   Due to alkalosis

16. a. True   Acid in the duodenum inactivates lipase leading to fat malabsorption
     b. False The acid output is already high due to high resting gastrin levels, and the extra pentagastrin makes little difference
     c. False
     d. False Complications of peptic ulceration are the main cause of death
     e. True   Especially parathyroid and adrenal

17. a. True   Thiamine deficiency in alcoholics commonly causes this
     b. False Will occur with portal hypertension of any cause
     c. True   Probably reflects malnutrition
     d. False Alcoholic cirrhosis is usually micronodular
     e. False This might raise another possible aetiology

18. a. True   And also with other thrombotic disorders
     b. False The jugular venous pulse is dissociated from the liver by the obstruction. Hepatojugular reflux is negative. Giant 'v' waves are a feature of tricuspid incompetence
     c. False Classically there is increased uptake centrally over the caudate lobe, because it drains separately into the inferior vena cava
     d. True
     e. False Gross hepatic venous congestion dominates

19. **In a case of malabsorption a histologically normal peroral jejunal biopsy would be against the diagnosis of—**
    a. Dermatitis herpetiformis
    b. Intestinal lymphangiectasia
    c. Crohn's disease
    d. Whipple's disease
    e. Lactase deficiency

20. **Characteristic features of vitamin C deficiency include—**
    a. Low output of ascorbic acid in the urine after a large oral load
    b. Pigmented rash on the light exposed areas
    c. Perifollicular haemorrhages
    d. Heart failure
    e. Peripheral neuropathy

Answers overleaf

19. a. True At least some degree of villous atrophy is usual
 b. True Characteristically dilated lymphatics in the lamina propria are seen
 c. False Crohn's disease causes malabsorption by a variety of mechanisms. Only a limited section of small intestine may be involved
 d. True PAS positive macrophages in the lamina propria are typical
 e. False The mucosa is grossly normal. Enzyme assays are required for diagnosis

20. a. True The deficient tissues avidly take up ascorbic acid
 b. False This is typical of pellagra
 c. True
 d. False This is typical of beri-beri
 e. False Again a feature of beri-beri

Genetics

1. **Autosomal recessive inheritance is found in—**
   a. Hunter's syndrome
   b. Galactosaemia
   c. von Gierke's disease
   d. Tuberous sclerosis
   e. Huntingdon's chorea

2. **In sex-linked recessive inheritance—**
   a. Only males are affected
   b. All the sisters of an affected male are usually carriers
   c. Approximately half the brothers of carrier females will have the disease
   d. The parents of an affected male are usually outwardly normal
   e. Half the sons of affected males will have the disease

3. **Sex-linked inheritance is found in—**
   a. Osteogenesis imperfecta
   b. Vitamin-D-resistant rickets
   c. Limb girdle muscular dystrophy
   d. Christmas disease
   e. Glucose-6-phosphate dehydrogenase deficiency

4. **Abnormalities of chromosomes are a feature of—**
   a. Testicular feminisation syndrome
   b. Chronic myeloid leukaemia
   c. Turner's syndrome
   d. Fanconi's aplastic anaemia
   e. Marfan's syndrome

5. **Characteristic features of Klinefelter's syndrome include—**
   a. Low levels of gonadotrophins
   b. Impotence
   c. Gynaecomastia
   d. Short stature
   e. Congenital heart defects

Answers overleaf

1. a. False   It is sex-linked, unlike the other mucopolysacchar-idoses which have autosomal recessive inheritance
   b. True   Most of the disorders involving enzyme defects have autosomal recessive inheritance. In this case it is galactose-1-phosphate uridyl transferase
   c. True   Glucose-6-phosphatase is deficient
   d. False   Autosomal dominant
   e. False   Autosomal dominant

2. a. False   Beware only and never. An affected male may marry a carrier female and his daughters may have the disease
   b. False   About half his sisters will be carriers
   c. True   Though some female carriers could have new muta-tions. But to answer 'false' on this basis would be complicating the issue too much
   d. True
   e. False   None will have it

3. a. False   Usually autosomal dominant
   b. True   One of the few examples of sex-linked dominant inheritance
   c. False   Autosomal recessive
   d. True   Like factor VIII deficiency, it is sex-linked recessive
   e. True

4. a. False   A normal male karyotype is found
   b. True   The Philadelphia chromosome results from translocation
   c. True   45 X0 is the usual karyotype
   d. True   Various chromosomal abnormalities may be found
   e. False   Autosomal dominant inheritance is found

5. a. False   They are high due to feedback from a low testosterone
   b. False   Though they are generally infertile
   c. True
   d. False   They are often tall
   e. False   This is a feature of Turner's syndrome

Haematology

1. In a patient newly diagnosed as chronic myeloid leukaemia characteristic features would include—
    a. Thrombocytopenia
    b. Basophilia
    c. Reduced leucocyte alkaline phosphatase
    d. Low B_{12}
    e. Elevated uric acid

2. Disorders in which there is an abnormal amino acid substitution in the haemoglobin polypeptide chain include—
    a. Paroxysmal nocturnal haemoglobinuria
    b. Methaemoglobinaemia
    c. Sickle cell trait
    d. Glucose-6-phosphate dehydrogenase deficiency
    e. α-thalassaemia

3. A myeloid type of leukaemoid reaction is recognised with—
    a. Subphrenic abscess
    b. Carcinoma of the lung with bone metastases
    c. Infectious mononucleosis
    d. Acute haemolysis
    e. Whooping cough

4. Indications for splenectomy include—
    a. Polycythaemia vera rubra
    b. Chronic idiopathic thrombocytopenic purpura
    c. Auto-immune haemolytic anaemia
    d. Felty's syndrome
    e. Pernicious anaemia

Answers overleaf

1. a. False   Normal or increased platelet numbers are present in the early stages
    b. True
    c. True   It may increase at the stage of blast cell transformation
    d. False   It is characteristically elevated
    e. True   Though clinical gout is not a common presenting feature

2. a. False   A red cell membrane defect is the problem
    b. False   This is where haem is oxidised to the ferric state, and is drug- or chemical-induced usually
    c. True   Valine is substituted for glutamic acid at the sixth position of the β-chain
    d. False
    e. False   Due to the failure of synthesis of α-chains, γ and β chains are present in excess, but this is not the result of amino acid substitution

3. a. True   As with other infections producing a profound neutrophil leucocytosis
    b. True
    c. False   The blood picture is more likely to be confused with lymphatic leukaemia
    d. True
    e. False   A marked lymphocytosis may be seen

4. a. False
    b. True   Though splenomegaly is not prominent
    c. True   The spleen is usually the main site of red blood cell destruction
    d. True   Where hypersplenism is a problem
    e. False   Splenomegaly, which is found in less than 10 per cent of cases, subsides with adequate replacement

5. **Haemolytic disorders in which haemolysis is characteristically intravascular include—**
   a. β-thalassaemia
   b. Hereditary spherocytosis
   c. Paroxysmal nocturnal haemoglobinuria
   d. Blackwater fever
   e. Pyruvate kinase deficiency

6. **Characteristic features of chronic idiopathic thrombocytopenic purpura include—**
   a. Females more often affected than males
   b. Bleeding into joints
   c. Splenomegaly
   d. Decreased number of mega-karyocytes in the bone marrow
   e. Prolonged bleeding time

7. **Increased serum iron is a feature of—**
   a. Anaemia due to chronic infection
   b. Thalassaemia
   c. Sideroblastic anaemia
   d. Haemochromatosis
   e. Pernicious anaemia

8. **A dimorphic blood picture is a feature of—**
   a. Sideroblastic anaemia
   b. Malabsorption
   c. Thalassaemia
   d. Recent blood transfusion
   e. Aplastic anaemia

Answers overleaf

5. a. False
    b. False   Extravascular haemolysis is usual for most haemolytic anaemias with red cells being destroyed in the spleen
    c. True   The classic case of intravascular haemolysis. It also occurs in heart valve haemolysis, mis-matched transfusions, infections, burns and sometimes in auto-immune haemolytic anaemia and glucose-6-phosphate dehydrogenase deficiency
    d. True   *Clostridium whelchii* septicaemia is the other typical infective cause
    e. False

6. a. True   In the acute type sex incidence is equal
    b. False   Bleeding into the skin and mucous membranes is typical as with other platelet disorders
    c. False   This occurs in only 10% and is slight
    d. False   Mega-karyocytes are normal or increased. The problem is increased platelet destruction due to circulating antibodies
    e. True   As with any marked thrombocytopenia

7. a. False   Low iron with low iron-binding capacity is usual. Note that in general serum iron can be unreliable, and serum ferretin is a better indicator of iron stores
    b. True   Iron overload is a serious complication
    c. True   Due to failure of iron utilisation
    d. True
    e. True   It falls rapidly with treatment

8. a. True   Both normochromic and hypochromic cells are found
    b. True   Due to mixed iron and folate/B_{12} deficiency
    c. False
    d. True   Liver disease is the other main cause of a dimorphic picture due to oesophageal bleeding plus folate deficiency
    e. False

9. **Thrombocytopenia is a recognised feature of—**
   a. von Willebrand's disease
   b. Systemic lupus erythematosus
   c. Henoch–Schönlein purpura
   d. Wiskott–Aldrich syndrome
   e. Disseminated intravascular coagulation

10. **A microcytic blood picture is seen in—**
   a. β-thalassaemia minor
   b. Scurvy
   c. Sideroblastic anaemia
   d. Chronic lead poisoning
   e. Pyruvate-kinase deficiency

11. **Characteristic features of von Willebrand's disease include—**
   a. Sex-linked inheritance
   b. Disordered platelet aggregation
   c. Prolonged prothrombin time
   d. Correction of bleeding tendency by administration of serum from haemophiliacs
   e. Bleeding into large joints

12. **A patient has a monoclonal paraprotein band on electrophoresis. Indications that it represents malignant disease include—**
   a. Bence–Jones protein in the urine
   b. Paraprotein of IgG class
   c. Depression of other immunoglobulin fractions
   d. Presence of lytic bone lesions
   e. Paraprotein level of 30 g/l

13. **Eosinophilia in the peripheral blood is characteristic of—**
   a. Schistosomiasis
   b. Kala-azar
   c. Rubella
   d. Hypothyroidism
   e. Asthma

Answers overleaf

9. a. False Though platelet function is disturbed
b. True Occasionally this is the presenting feature
c. False
d. True A sex-linked syndrome including eczema and depressed immunity
e. True

10. a. True
b. False It is normocytic or occasionally slightly macrocytic
c. True
d. True Haem synthesis is reduced due to block in porphyrin metabolism
e. False

11. a. False It is autosomal dominant
b. True
c. False The defect is in the intrinsic clotting system, producing a prolonged partial thromboplastin time
d. True
e. False Bleeding into mucous membranes and skin is more usual. Contrast haemophilia

12. a. True
b. False The benign peaks are usually IgG, though IgG peaks can of course be malignant
c. True
d. True
e. True Very high levels and a rising level of paraprotein point towards malignant disease

13. a. True As with many other parasitic infestations
b. False A leucopenia is usual
c. False
d. False Basophilia occasionally occurs
e. True Remember polyarteritis nodosa, Hodgkin's and allergies as the other main causes of eosinophilia

14. **Spherocytes in the peripheral blood are seen in—**
    a. Auto-immune haemolytic anaemia
    b. Hereditary spherocytosis
    c. Multiple myeloma
    d. Severe burns
    e. Lead poisoning

15. **Clinically detectable splenomegaly is characteristic of—**
    a. Hereditary spherocytosis
    b. Sickle cell disease in an adult
    c. β-thalassaemia major
    d. Glucose-6-phosphate dehydrogenase deficiency
    e. Auto-immune haemolytic anaemia

16. **A neutrophil leucocytosis is characteristic of—**
    a. Influenza
    b. Leptospirosis
    c. Diphtheria
    d. Typhoid
    e. Pertussis

17. **A 55-year-old man has massive splenomegaly. Features which suggest chronic myeloid leukaemia rather than myelofibrosis include—**
    a. A white cell count greater than 50,000 per mm^3 (50×10^9/l)
    b. Elevated neutrophil alkaline phosphatase
    c. Frequent nucleated red blood cells in the peripheral blood
    d. Presence of Philadelphia chromosome
    e. Anaemia

Answers overleaf

14. a. True   Hereditary spherocytosis is not the only cause. Spherocytes are produced as a result of auto-immune haemolysis
    b. True   Here spherocytosis is the cause of haemolysis
    c. False
    d. True
    e. False

15. a. True
    b. False   By adult life the spleen is shrunken from repeated infarction
    c. True
    d. False   Splenomegaly is not prominent
    e. True

16. a. False   Significant leucocytosis might suggest secondary bacterial infection
    b. True   Helpful in distinguishing the causes of hepatitis
    c. True
    d. False   Leucopenia is usual. A sudden leucocytosis might suggest a perforation
    e. False   Lymphocytosis is characteristic

17. a. True   The white cell count may be elevated in myelofibrosis but rarely to that degree
    b. False   It is low in chronic myeloid. In myelofibrosis it is normal or increased
    c. False   Primitive red cells are typical of myelofibrosis
    d. True
    e. False   Anaemia occurs in both

18. **Features of polycythaemia vera rubra include—**
    a. Reduced plasma volume
    b. Haemorrhagic tendency
    c. Elevated ESR
    d. Pruritus
    e. Increased neutrophil alkaline phosphatase

19. **An attack of acute intermittent porphyria is characterised by—**
    a. Diarrhoea
    b. Confusion
    c. Hypotension
    d. Bullous rash
    e. Abdominal pain

20. **Characteristic features of porphyria cutanea tarda include—**
    a. An association with alcohol abuse
    b. Neurological symptoms
    c. Need for iron supplements
    d. Photosensitivity
    e. Increased urinary porphobilinogen

Answers overleaf

18. a. False The plasma volume is normal. The red cell volume is increased and therefore the total blood volume is increased
    b. True   Surgery is a particular hazard. Vascular engorgement and platelet abnormalities are two contributory factors to the bleeding tendency
    c. False It is rarely greater than 1 mm in the first hour
    d. True   Histamine release is thought to be responsible
    e. True

19. a. False Constipation is usual
    b. True   A variety of psychiatric manifestations are seen
    c. False Hypertension and tachycardia are usual
    d. False Skin problems are not a feature of this type of porphyria
    e. True

20. a. True   Excess alcohol and an enzyme defect are probably the main factors in causation
    b. False Unlike acute intermittent porphyria
    c. False Iron overload is the rule. Venesection is standard treatment
    d. True
    e. False These are hard to remember, but this is the finding in acute intermittent porphyria

Immunology

1. **Circulating immune complexes are important in the pathogenesis of —**
   a. Goodpasture's syndrome
   b. Pernicious anaemia
   c. Nephrotic syndrome due to malaria
   d. Serum sickness
   e. Allergic rhinitis

2. **Of disorders causing immunodeficiency, those affecting predominantly the cell mediated system include —**
   a. The di George syndrome
   b. Protein calorie malnutrition
   c. Chronic lymphatic leukaemia
   d. Sarcoidosis
   e. Nephrotic syndrome

3. **Chronic granulomatous disease is characterised by —**
   a. Inability of neutrophils to phagocytose bacteria
   b. Chronically enlarged lymph nodes
   c. Recurrent candidiasis
   d. Dominant inheritance
   e. Hypogammaglobulinaemia

4. **IgM —**
   a. Crosses the placenta
   b. Is a potent activator of complement
   c. Is the predominant immunoglobulin elevated in chronic active hepatitis
   d. Is produced after the other immunoglobulins in response to infection
   e. Is the predominant immunoglobulin involved in warm type auto-immune haemolytic anaemia

Answers overleaf

1. a. False Antibodies react directly with the glomerular base-
ment membrane, being deposited in a linear fashion,
in contrast to the lumpy deposition of immune
complex nephritis
   b. False Again autoantibodies seem to be directly involved
   c. True   A number of other infective agents also act as antigens in immune complex nephritis
   d. True
   e. False An example of type I hypersensitivity

2. a. True   There is failure of thymic development and hence the
T-lymphocytes
   b. True   Although humoral immunity is also depressed
   c. False Humoral immunity is predominantly affected due to
hypogammaglobulinaemia
   d. True   Remember the negative Mantoux test
   e. False Erysipelas and pneumococcal peritonitis were common
terminal events in the pre-antibiotic era. Defence
against these agents is largely antibody mediated

3. a. False The problem is inability to kill ingested bacteria
   b. True   They may suppurate, break down and form sinuses
   c. False Bacteria such as staphylococci and Gram-negative
species predominate
   d. False It is probably sex-linked
   e. False Gammaglobulins may be elevated in response to
chronic infection

4. a. False IgG is the main immunoglobulin which crosses the
placenta
   b. True   Due to the many binding sites for antigen
   c. False It is IgG
   d. False It is the first immunoglobulin produced
   e. False IgM is responsible for the cold type, except paroxysmal cold haemoglobinuria

5. **Tests directed at assessment of the cell-mediated immune system include—**

   a. Skin test with streptokinase/streptodornase
   b. Nitro-blue tetrazolium test
   c. Response of lymphocytes to phytohaemagglutinin
   d. Counting the lymphocytes which form rosettes with sheep red cells
   e. Measuring complement levels

Answers overleaf

5. a. True A number of other antigens (e.g. tuberculin, candida) are also used in skin testing
   b. False Defective polymorph function is indicated by failure to reduce nitro-blue tetrazolium
   c. True The proliferation of T-lymphocytes in response to this is measured
   d. True This identifies T-lymphocytes
   e. False

Infectious and Tropical Diseases

1. **The rash of measles characteristically —**
   a. Indicates the cessation of infectivity once it appears
   b. Spares the face
   c. Begins on the trunk
   d. Appears at the time of maximum fever
   e. Begins 1–2 days after the appearance of Koplik's spots

2. **Recognised complications of chicken pox include —**
   a. Pancreatitis
   b. Cerebellar ataxia
   c. Thrombocytopenia
   d. Viral pneumonia especially in adults
   e. Erythema marginatum

3. **Characteristically the rash of typhoid fever —**
   a. Appears in the first week of the illness
   b. Is worst on the face and limbs
   c. Lasts about 10 days
   d. Blanches on pressure
   e. Itches intensely

4. **Cryptococcus neoformans —**
   a. Is a filamentous fungi
   b. Complicates lymphomas
   c. Is characteristically found in soil contaminated by pigeon droppings
   d. Produces symptoms in the respiratory system most commonly
   e. Is resistant to known antifungal agents

5. **Recognised presentations of taenia solium infestation include —**
   a. Urticarial rash
   b. Epilepsy
   c. Macrocytic anaemia
   d. Liver abscess
   e. Weight loss

Answers overleaf

1. a. False Although the catarrhal phase is the period of maximal infectivity
   b. False
   c. False It begins at the hairline and behind the ears typically
   d. False Maximum fever is at the onset of the illness. The rash does not appear for 3–4 days
   e. True

2. a. False It does complicate certain virus infections, typically mumps
   b. True Due to encephalitis
   c. True Occasionally it causes bleeding into the skin lesions
   d. True The pneumonia in adults can be serious
   e. False

3. a. False The second week
   b. False It is worst on the trunk
   c. False It usually lasts 2–3 days
   d. True
   e. False

4. a. False It is a yeast and unlike some other yeasts cannot change to a mycelium
   b. True Immunosuppression predisposes to many fungal infections
   c. True Rich nitrogen content is ideal for fungal survival
   d. False Neurological symptoms and signs are most common
   e. False Amphotericin is quite effective

5. a. True At the stage of larval invasion
   b. True
   c. False Do not confuse *Diphyllobothrium latum*
   d. False Do not confuse hydatid disease
   e. True A symptom of adult worm infestation

6. Recognised features of *Schistosoma mansoni* infestation include—
   a. Reliable diagnosis by rectal biopsy
   b. Interstitial pulmonary fibrosis
   c. Immune complex nephrotic syndrome
   d. Splenomegaly
   e. Diarrhoea

7. Characteristic features of tuberculoid leprosy include—
   a. Positive lepromin test
   b. Isolation of organisms from the skin
   c. Symmetrical peripheral neuropathy
   d. Negligible risk of person-to-person spread
   e. Iritis

8. The following infections characteristically have an incubation period of less than seven days—
   a. Scarlet fever
   b. Measles
   c. Cholera
   d. Typhoid
   e. Brucellosis

9. Characteristic features of infectious mononucleosis include—
   a. Anaemia
   b. Sore throat
   c. Petechiae on the soft palate
   d. White cell count of 50,000 per mm^3 (50 × 10^9/l)
   e. Splenomegaly

10. Characteristic features of yellow fever include—
    a. A relative bradycardia accompanying fever
    b. Transmission by lice
    c. Centrizonal necrosis of the liver
    d. Bleeding tendency
    e. Good response to penicillin

Answers overleaf

6. a. True
   b. True   When eggs bypass the liver via portacaval anastomoses
   c. True
   d. True   Due to portal hypertension
   e. True   Due to bowel involvement

7. a. True   Due to well developed hypersensitivity
   b. False   Unlike lepromatous leprosy
   c. False   This is typical of lepromatous leprosy. In tuberculoid, nerves, e.g. greater auricular, are singled out here and there
   d. True   The risk is greater in lepromatous leprosy
   e. False   A feature of lepromatous leprosy

8. a. True   2–5 days
   b. False   7–14 days
   c. True   Usually a few hours
   d. False   7–21 days
   e. False   7–28 days

9. a. False   Anaemia, lymphadenopathy and abnormal lymphocytes would suggest leukaemia. However, rarely a haemolytic anaemia is recognised in infectious mononucleosis
   b. True
   c. True
   d. False   Leucocytosis of this degree should suggest the possibility of leukaemia
   e. True

10. a. True   Faget's sign
    b. False   Mosquitoes are involved
    c. False   Midzonal necrosis, which is also seen in Lassa fever occurs
    d. True
    e. False   An arbo virus is the cause, which is not penicillin sensitive

11. **A bleeding tendency is a recognised feature of—**
    a. Leptospirosis
    b. Poliomyelitis
    c. Ebola virus disease
    d. Cholera
    e. Yellow fever

12. **There is negligible risk of person-to-person spread of infection in—**
    a. Marburg virus disease
    b. Mumps once salivary gland swelling appears
    c. Brucellosis
    d. Measles once the rash appears
    e. Varicella before the rash appears

13. ***Clostridium tetani*—**
    a. Is a Gram-negative bacillus
    b. Forms spores easily
    c. Invades the nervous system
    d. Can be killed effectively by administration of antiserum
    e. Causes most severe illness following a very short incubation period

14. **Features of Legionnaires' disease include—**
    a. Causation by DNA virus
    b. Most severe course in young fit individuals
    c. Rapid person-to-person spread
    d. Peak incidence in summer
    e. Mental confusion

15. **Recognised features of cytomegalovirus infection include—**
    a. Markedly increased incidence of congenital heart defects in infants born to mothers with the disease
    b. Positive Paul–Bunnell test
    c. Purpura
    d. Increased incidence in renal dialysis patients
    e. Hepatosplenomegaly

Answers overleaf

11. a. True   Due to liver disease
    b. False
    c. True   Probably due to disseminated intravascular coagulation
    d. False
    e. True

12. a. False   Contact with blood, urine and semen of infected cases causes the disease
    b. False   Although the maximal infectivity is before swelling occurs
    c. True   Person-to-person spread is very rare
    d. False   Infectivity persists for about another 4 days
    e. False   It is infectious for about 5 days before

13. a. False   It is Gram-positive
    b. True   Hence its ability to survive
    c. False   It is the toxin which affects the nervous system
    d. False   Antiserum neutralises the toxin
    e. True

14. a. False   A Gram-negative cocco-bacillus is responsible
    b. False   Fatality occurs in the old and infirm
    c. False   Present knowledge blames water and air-conditioning systems
    d. True
    e. True

15. a. False   Unlike congenital rubella
    b. False   Although like glandular fever atypical mononuclears are seen
    c. True   A feature of congenital CMV infection
    d. True   In such immunosuppressed patients disseminated infection is seen
    e. True

16. **Brucellosis—**
    a. Is a notifiable disease
    b. Produces agglutinins which may persist long after clinical recovery
    c. Is best treated with benzyl penicillin
    d. Is most commonly acquired by drinking infected milk
    e. Is characterised by a relative lymphocytosis

17. **Characteristic features of diphtheria include—**
    a. Incubation period of less than 7 days
    b. Spread by droplet infection
    c. Little benefit from the administration of antitoxin
    d. Most marked toxin formation when primary infection is in the nose
    e. A latent period of 2–8 weeks before neurological complications

18. **Features more typical of *Shigella* dysentery than typhoid include—**
    a. Chronic carrier state
    b. Growth of the causative organism in DCA (desoxycholate citrate) media
    c. Diagnosis by blood culture
    d. Bloody diarrhoea
    e. Leucocytosis

19. **In a patient with meningitis particular suspicion that the organism is a pneumococcus is raised if there is history of—**
    a. Feeling poorly with headaches for some weeks
    b. Chronic ear infection
    c. Sudden onset of the illness in a fit young army recruit
    d. Ventriculo-venous shunt for control of hydrocephalus
    e. Previous splenectomy

Answers overleaf

16. a. False
     b. True   Thus difficulty may arise in differentiating those with acute illness from those with previous exposure
     c. False   Tetracyclines are the usual choice
     d. False   With pasteurisation of milk, infection is more often acquired by contact with diseased animals themselves
     e. True   The total white cell count is normal or slightly reduced

17. a. True
     b. True
     c. False   Since its use mortality has fallen dramatically
     d. False   Oropharyngeal involvement is associated with maximum toxin formation
     e. True   Although cranial nerve lesions may occur earlier

18. a. False   Carriage of *Shigella* is rare. Numerous infamous typhoid carriers are well documented
     b. False   Both grow well on this
     c. False   Septicaemia is rare with *Shigella*
     d. True   In typhoid constipation is usual
     e. True   Slight leucocytosis is common while in typhoid leucopenia is usual

19. a. False   Typical of tuberculous meningitis
     b. True
     c. False   This would be typical of meningococcal meningitis
     d. False   *Staphylococcus albus* is a particularly common cause of meningitis in these patients, although it is normally a skin commensal
     e. True   Particularly in younger patients the incidence of infection is increased after splenectomy. The pneumococcus is one of the commonest organisms involved

20. **Drug prophylaxis for malaria—**

    a. Is required when travelling to parts of South America

    b. Is unnecessary for those born in malarial areas, but resident in Britain, who go home for holidays

    c. Can cease a few days after leaving a malarial area

    d. With chloroquine is unsatisfactory in most parts of Africa due to drug resistance

    e. Is advisable for a person living in a malarial area moving to another distant malarial area.

Answers overleaf

20. a. True Many parts are still malarial
    b. False Immunity drops in those resident in non-malarial areas
    c. False It should continue for 4 weeks so that parasites which continue to be released from the liver can be destroyed
    d. False Chloroquine resistance is commonest in South-East Asia and South America
    e. True Different strains and different immunity may be involved

Microbiology

1. **Organisms that are Gram-positive include—**
    a. *Bordetella pertussis*
    b. *Corynebacterium diphtheriae*
    c. *Clostridium welchii*
    d. *Bacillus anthracis*
    e. *Shigella sonnei*

2. **Antibiotics that act predominantly by interference with the bacterial cell wall include—**
    a. Benzyl penicillin
    b. Streptomycin
    c. Tetracycline
    d. Actinomycin
    e. Cephaloridin

3. **A previously fit boy of 16 develops pneumonia. Organisms likely to be responsible include—**
    a. *Haemophilus influenzae*
    b. *Mycoplasma pneumoniae*
    c. *Pneumococcus*
    d. *Staphylococcus aureus*
    e. *Pseudomonas aeruginosa*

4. **Neisseria meningitidis—**
    a. Is a Gram-negative bacillus
    b. Can be found inside polymorphs in the CSF in patients with meningitis
    c. May produce chronic infection lasting some months characterised by rashes and arthralgia
    d. Is spread mainly by asymptomatic nasopharyngeal carriers
    e. Causes meningitis most commonly in young army recruits

Answers overleaf

1. a. False   It is a Gram-negative cocco-bacillus
   b. True   A Gram-positive rod
   c. True   A Gram-positive bacillus
   d. True   A Gram-positive bacillus
   e. False   It is a Gram-negative bacillus

2. a. True   Synthesis of cell wall mucopeptide is inhibited
   b. False   The main effect is on protein synthesis, which in turn causes reduced cellular respiration and nucleic acid turnover
   c. False   This also interferes with protein synthesis and prevents binding of transfer RNA to ribosomes
   d. False   It complexes with DNA and prevents nucleic acid synthesis. It is usually used against tumour cells rather than bacteria
   e. True   The cephalosporins have a similar mode of action to the penicillins

3. a. False   It usually causes infection secondary to pre-existing chronic bronchitis
   b. True   It is quite common amongst young people in closed institutions. It is rare above the age of 40
   c. True   Classic lobar pneumonia is less common. The pneumococcus is also common in exacerbations of chronic bronchitis
   d. False   Infection usually occurs as a complication of existing lung disease (e.g. cystic fibrosis) or influenza
   e. False   Pneumonia due to *Pseudomonas* usually occurs in hospital in debilitated or immuno-suppressed patients

4. a. False   They are oval cocci arranged in pairs
   b. True   The intracellular location is typical
   c. True   Such chronic meningococcaemia is uncommon
   d. True   Only small numbers in the population will get the disease, but 5–10 per cent are carriers
   e. False   It is commonest in infants. A second lower peak occurs in young adults in closed communities

5. **Viruses of which the nucleic acid core consists of DNA include—**
   a. Herpes zoster virus
   b. Togaviruses
   c. Adenovirus
   d. Poliovirus
   e. Influenza virus

Answers overleaf

5. a. True   As are other members of the herpes virus group, e.g. cytomegalovirus, Epstein–Barr virus and herpes simplex
    b. False Formerly called the 'arboviruses', this group (including the yellow fever virus) has an RNA core
    c. True
    d. False The enteroviruses, of which poliovirus is one, are RNA viruses
    e. False The myxoviruses, of which influenza is one, are RNA viruses

Neurology

1. Recognised features of lesions of the frontal lobe include—
    a. Astereognosis
    b. Positive grasp reflex
    c. Superior homonymous quadrantanopia
    d. Unilateral optic atrophy
    e. Anosmia

2. Factors associated with the development of migraine headache include—
    a. Age over 70 years
    b. Oral contraception
    c. History of abdominal upset in childhood
    d. Intracerebral angioma
    e. Hypertension

3. Calcification on skull X-ray is found in—
    a. Jakob-Creutzfeldt disease
    b. Craniopharyngioma
    c. Hypoparathyroidism
    d. Herpes simplex encephalitis
    e. Chronic subdural haematoma

4. In post-encephalitic Parkinsonism—
    a. Oculogyric crises are characteristic
    b. Signs of hypothalamic damage are recognised
    c. Somnolence is characteristic
    d. The onset is earlier than in idiopathic Parkinsonism
    e. Tremor is especially prominent

5. Characteristic features of myotonia congenita include—
    a. Worsening with exposure to heat
    b. Improvement after repeated voluntary activity
    c. Persistence after curarisation
    d. Fasciculation in the affected muscle
    e. Involvement of the long flexors of the hands

Answers overleaf

1. a. False This is characteristic of parietal lobe lesions
    b. True
    c. False This is a feature of temporal lobe lesions
    d. True   This may be produced by pressure on the optic nerve.
               Associated with increased intracranial pressure papill-
               oedema may occur in the other eye. This is called
               the Foster-Kennedy syndrome
    e. True   The olfactory nerve lies beneath the frontal lobe

2. a. False The onset is usually in young people
    b. True   If migraine occurs the pill should be stopped
    c. True
    d. True
    e. False

3. a. False
    b. True   Look just above the pituitary fossa
    c. True   Calcification in the basal ganglia is found in about
               half these patients
    d. False
    e. True   The organised clot may eventually calcify

4. a. True   They are also common in drug-induced Parkinsonism
    b. True   For example sweating and hypersalivation
    c. False This is characteristic of the precipitating illness—
               encephalitis lethargica
    d. True
    e. False

5. a. False Cold usually exacerbates
    b. True
    c. True   The defect is in the muscle membrane
    d. False
    e. True   The tongue is also very commonly affected

6. **Characteristic features of motor neurone disease include—**
   a. Fasciculation
   b. Hesitancy of micturition
   c. Early loss of abdominal reflexes
   d. Nystagmus
   e. Intellectual deterioration

7. **Characteristic features of Wilson's disease include—**
   a. Raised serum copper
   b. Amino-aciduria
   c. Autosomal dominant inheritance
   d. Onset in the first year of life
   e. Haemolytic anaemia

8. **A prolapsed intervertebral disc between L4 and L5 vertebrae can produce on the affected side—**
   a. An absent knee jerk
   b. Impaired dorsiflexion of the foot
   c. Reduced sensation over the great toe
   d. An absent ankle jerk
   e. Reduced straight leg raising

9. **Characteristic causes of a predominantly motor peripheral neuropathy include—**
   a. Lead poisoning
   b. Diphtheria
   c. B_{12} deficiency
   d. Leprosy
   e. Guillain-Barré syndrome

10. **Ptosis is a recognised feature of—**
    a. Friedreich's ataxia
    b. Wilson's disease
    c. Dystrophia myotonica
    d. Occlusion of the posterior inferior cerebellar artery
    e. Salbutamol therapy

Answers overleaf

6. a. True   Fasciculation occurs in lower motor neurone lesions, especially when damage is near the anterior horn cell
    b. False Urinary problems are late
    c. False These may be preserved until late, unlike multiple sclerosis where they are lost early
    d. False Oddly the ocular nuclei are spared
    e. False The intellect may be intact to the end

7. a. False It is low due to low levels of the binding protein caeruloplasmin
    b. True   Phosphate is also lost in the urine and may lead to bone disease
    c. False It is recessive
    d. False Between 6 and 20 years would be typical
    e. True

8. a. False Between L4 and L5 vertebrae the affected nerve root is L5. The knee jerk is controlled by roots L3 and L4
    b. True   This movement is controlled by roots L4 and L5
    c. True
    d. False The ankle jerk is controlled by S1 and S2 roots
    e. True

9. a. True   For example the painter's wrist drop
    b. True   Remember the respiratory paralysis
    c. False There are prominent sensory findings as well
    d. False
    e. True   The other predominant motor neuropathy is acute intermittent porphyria

10. a. False
    b. False
    c. True
    d. True   Due to interruption of the sympathetic supply in the lateral medulla
    e. False Sympathetic stimulation causes lid retraction

11. **In chronic subdural haematoma—**
    a. Men are more often affected than women
    b. Lumbar puncture is essential
    c. An association with alcohol abuse is recognised
    d. A history of progressive dementia over some years is characteristic
    e. An isotope brain scan is a useful diagnostic test

12. **Characteristic features of temporal lobe epilepsy include—**
    a. 3 per second spike and wave pattern on the electro-encephalogram
    b. A better response to drug therapy than with other types of epilepsy
    c. Olfactory hallucinations
    d. Outbursts of antisocial behaviour
    e. Seizures beginning with a localised group of muscles and then spreading to others

13. **Causes of cerebellar ataxia include—**
    a. Motor neurone disease
    b. Chronic alcoholism
    c. Phenytoin
    d. Wilson's disease
    e. Bronchial carcinoma

14. **Cauda equina lesions characteristically produce—**
    a. Hyperreflexia of the lower limbs
    b. Impotence
    c. Loss of abdominal reflexes
    d. Sensory loss over saddle area of the buttocks
    e. Loss of tone of the anal sphincter

Answers overleaf

11. a. True
    b. False   It is avoided because of the risk of coning
    c. True
    d. False   The history is rarely longer than a few months
    e. True

12. a. False   This is characteristic of *petit mal* epilepsy
    b. False   Good control of seizures is often difficult
    c. True   As well as other types of hallucination
    d. True
    e. False   This would be typical of an epileptic focus near
               the motor cortex

13. a. False
    b. True   As part of Wernicke's encephalopathy
    c. True
    d. False   The basal ganglia are affected
    e. True   Due either to secondaries or a non-metastatic effect

14. a. False   The cauda equina contains lower motor neurones
    b. True
    c. False   This would reflect an upper motor neurone lesion
    d. True   The area supplied by the sacral nerve roots
    e. True

15. Characteristic features of a lesion in the lateral part of the medulla include—

    a. Ipsilateral Horner's syndrome
    b. Contralateral loss of proprioception to the body and limbs
    c. Nystagmus
    d. Ipsilateral palsy of the hypoglossal nerve
    e. Dysphagia

16. Characteristic features of infective polyneuritis (Guillain-Barré syndrome) include—

    a. Pathological changes in the distal parts of the peripheral nerve
    b. Incontinence
    c. Sparing of cranial nerves
    d. Marked improvement with ACTH
    e. High pyrexia

17. Recognised features of myasthenia gravis include—

    a. Asymmetrical weakness
    b. An association with thyrotoxicosis
    c. Dysphagia
    d. Absent reflexes
    e. Sluggish pupillary responses

18. In facio-scapulo-humeral muscular dystrophy—

    a. Inheritance is autosomal dominant
    b. The patient usually needs a wheelchair by age 20
    c. Tendon reflexes are lost early
    d. CPK may be normal
    e. Winging of the scapulae is characteristic

Answers overleaf

15. a. True
    b. False   The medial lemniscus carrying proprioception is sited medially in the medulla
    c. True
    d. False   The twelfth nerve nucleus is sited medially
    e. True   Due to involvement of the ninth and tenth nerves

16. a. False   It is primarily a radiculopathy with changes in the nerve root
    b. False
    c. False   They are commonly involved
    d. False   The effect is debatable
    e. False   Low-grade pyrexia is usual

17. a. True   Also some groups of muscles may be profoundly affected (e.g. extraocular) while others appear to be spared
    b. True   It is also associated with other auto-immune diseases including systemic lupus
    c. True
    d. False   Generally reflexes and muscle bulk are preserved, except perhaps in very longstanding cases
    e. True   Though they are usually normal

18. a. True
    b. False   The course is often quite benign
    c. False   Reflexes are often spared until late in myopathies
    d. True   Reflecting the less florid process
    e. True

19. **Characteristic findings in the CSF of a patient with multiple sclerosis include—**
   a. Positive Wassermann reaction
   b. Oligoclonal pattern of immunoglobulins on electrophoresis
   c. Total protein of 1·2 g/l (120 mg/100 ml)
   d. Increased white cells especially polymorphs
   e. Reduced plasma: CSF bromide ratio in the bromide partition test

20. **Cerebrospinal fluid with increased protein and reduced sugar is seen in—**
   a. Sarcoidosis
   b. Echo virus meningitis
   c. Meningeal carcinomatosis
   d. Tuberculous meningitis
   e. Amoebic meningo-encephalitis

Answers overleaf

19. a. False Paretic Lange curve with negative Wassermann is typical

      b. True

      c. False Some increase in protein is usual but not to this degree

      d. False Increased lymphocytes may be seen

      e. False This is a test for tuberculous meningitis. It is based on the increased permeability of the blood brain barrier to bromide

20. a. True

      b. False A few cases of viral meningitis may cause a reduction in sugar, e.g. mumps

      c. True

      d. True At first the sugar may be normal, but if the lumbar puncture is repeated later, the sugar is usually low

      e. True

Occupational Diseases

1. **In decompression sickness—**
   a. Osteoporosis after long exposure is recognised
   b. Pruritus is a characteristic symptom
   c. Paraplegia complicates severe cases
   d. Treatment is by prompt recompression
   e. Symptoms of the 'bends' take about 6 hours to develop

2. **Characteristic features of poisoning with tetraethyl lead include—**
   a. Colic
   b. Wrist drop
   c. Mental confusion
   d. Severe anaemia
   e. Rapid response of symptoms to EDTA

3. **There is a recognised risk of lung cancer associated with exposure to—**
   a. Tin
   b. Chromium
   c. Nickel
   d. Aluminium
   e. Uranium

4. **Characteristic features of chronic cadmium poisoning include—**
   a. Peripheral neuropathy
   b. Proteinuria
   c. Anosmia
   d. Emphysema
   e. Confusion

5. **Industrial injuries benefit under the Prescribed Diseases regulations may be claimed by—**
   a. A farmworker with brucellosis
   b. An aniline dye worker with gastric cancer
   c. A nurse with tuberculosis
   d. A flax worker with lung cancer
   e. A docker with a prolapsed intervertebral disc

Answers overleaf

1.   a.   False   Aseptic necrosis is the recognised bone complication
      b.   True
      c.   True
      d.   True
      e.   False   Usually they occur within the hour. The 'chokes' may take some hours to appear

2.   a.   False   The point is that the features of organic and inorganic lead poisoning are quite different. Colic is not a feature
      b.   False
      c.   True   This dominates thé picture. Acute mania is seen
      d.   False   Mild anaemia is a feature of inorganic lead poisoning
      e.   False   EDTA cannot bind triethyl lead, the prevalent metabolite of tetraethyl lead

3.   a.   False   Tin may give X-ray abnormalities, but appears to be harmless
      b.   True   Cancer of the nose also occurs
      c.   True
      d.   False   Fumes produce an acute respiratory disorder which is occasionally complicated by pneumothorax
      e.   True

4.   a.   False
      b.   True   The lesion seems to be in the renal tubules
      c.   True   With atrophy of the nasal mucosa
      d.   True
      e.   False

5.   a.   True   To apply, the disease must be one which is listed, and the occupation one where exposure to the risk has occurred
      b.   False   There is no association
      c.   True
      d.   False   Flax workers get byssinosis
      e.   False   Although a docker might acquire such a lesion in his work, a prolapsed disc is not a Prescribed Disease

Ophthalmology

1. **Causes of optic atrophy include—**

   a. Syphilis
   b. Motor neurone disease
   c. Friedreich's ataxia
   d. Isoniazid
   e. Syringomyelia

2. **Characteristic features of papilloedema include—**

   a. Pain behind the eye
   b. Early loss of vision
   c. Loss of light reflex
   d. Enlargement of the blind spot
   e. Loss of retinal venous pulsation

3. **Large pupils are a recognised feature of—**

   a. Holmes–Adie syndrome
   b. Third nerve palsy
   c. Horner's syndrome
   d. Poisoning with tricyclic antidepressants
   e. Motor neurone disease

4. **Anterior uveitis is a characteristic feature of—**

   a. Rheumatoid arthritis
   b. Sarcoidosis
   c. Thyrotoxicosis
   d. Reiter's syndrome
   e. Hypoparathyroidism

Answers overleaf

1. a. True   A classic finding in tabes, but also a feature of general paresis
    b. False   The optic nerve is a sensory nerve
    c. True   But is quite uncommon
    d. True   We tend to remember the peripheral neuropathy, but optic atrophy also occurs. Ethambutol also causes optic atrophy
    e. False

2. a. False   This is typical of optic neuritis and is helpful diagnostically, as papillitis may be hard to distinguish from papilloedema on ophthalmoscopy
    b. False   Loss of vision is a late feature, contrasting with optic neuritis
    c. False
    d. True   The blind spot results from the absence of photoreceptors over the optic nerve head. The size of the latter is increased by oedema
    e. True   This follows logically from the idea that increased intracranial pressure obstructs retinal venous drainage when it causes papilloedema

3. a. True   Occasionally. But the characteristic feature is its slow reaction to light
    b. True   Due to removal of the parasympathetic supply
    c. False   The parasympathetic supply now dominates
    d. True   Due to anticholinergic properties
    e. False   Oddly the ocular nuclei (3rd, 4th and 6th cranial nerves) are spared, so pupils and eye movements are normal

4. a. False   It is not characteristic. Scleritis is the typical finding
    b. True
    c. False
    d. True   As with other causes of seronegative arthritis
    e. False   Cataract is the usual ophthalmic problem

5. **Dry eyes are a recognised feature of—**
    a. Ankylosing spondylitis
    b. Riley–Day syndrome
    c. Practolol therapy
    d. Seventh nerve palsy
    e. Horner's syndrome

Answers overleaf

5. a. False   Dry eyes occur in Sjögren's syndrome which is usually associated with seropositive arthritis
    b. True   In this inherited disease the autonomic nervous system is disturbed and dry eyes are just one of many consequences
    c. True   A modern medical disaster
    d. True   Failure of lid closure allows drying
    e. False

Paediatrics

1. **Characteristic features of Fallot's tetralogy include—**
   a. Right axis shift on ECG
   b. Plethoric lung fields
   c. Loud pulmonary second sound
   d. Palliation by anastomosing the left subclavian artery to the pulmonary artery
   e. Systolic bruit due to ventricular septal defect

2. **Characteristic features of acute post-streptococcal glomerulonephritis include—**
   a. Dehydration
   b. Poor eventual prognosis
   c. Facial oedema
   d. Low serum complement levels
   e. Onset before 4 years of age

3. **Recognised features of congenital pyloric stenosis include—**
   a. Bile-stained vomiting
   b. Absence of nerve plexuses in the pyloric wall
   c. Conjugated hyperbilirubinaemia
   d. Greater incidence in males than females
   e. Palpable abdominal mass

4. **Findings recognised as normal in a 5-year-old child include the presence of—**
   a. Fixed splitting of the second heart sound
   b. A third heart sound
   c. A sound heard in the upper chest, in systole and diastole, which disappears when the neck veins are occluded
   d. An apical systolic thrill
   e. Elevated jugular venous pressure

Answers overleaf

1. a. True   Left axis shift in a child with cyanotic congenital heart disease raises the possibility of tricuspid atresia
    b. False   Flow to the pulmonary arteries is obstructed by right ventricular out-flow obstruction
    c. False   It is soft or inaudible
    d. True   This is Blalock's operation. Definitive repair is done earlier now and palliative operations are less often required
    e. False   The systolic bruit is usually due to subvalvular pulmonary stenosis

2. a. False   Fluid retention may lead to hypertension and cardiac failure
    b. False   A minority of experts feel that subsequent chronic renal disease is common. However, generally accepted teaching is that complete recovery usually occurs and that long-term sequelae are uncommon
    c. True
    d. True   Membrano-proliferative glomerulonephritis, systemic lupus, and infective endocarditis are the other main renal causes of low serum complement
    e. False   It usually occurs in school age children

3. a. False   The vomiting occurs during or shortly after feeding and may be projectile. Bile-stained vomiting would suggest obstruction at a lower level
    b. False   Nerve plexuses are absent from the intestinal wall in Hirschsprung's
    c. False   An unconjugated hyperbilirubinaemia is an occasional complication
    d. True
    e. True   The so-called 'pyloric tumour' can be felt during feeding in a relaxed infant

4. a. False   This is the typical finding with atrial septal defects
    b. True   This is recognised as physiological until the age of 30
    c. True   These features are characteristic of a venous hum
    d. False
    e. False

5. **In a neonate an unconjugated bilirubin of 120 mmol/l with little or no rise in the conjugated bilirubin is recognised in—**
   a. Rhesus incompatibility
   b. Dubin–Johnson syndrome
   c. Congenital biliary atresia
   d. Glucose-6-phosphate dehydrogenase deficiency
   e. Premature delivery

6. **Characteristically a child of 9 months can—**
   a. Grasp an object between finger and thumb
   b. Drink from a cup unaided
   c. Stand while holding onto support
   d. Comprehend simple commands
   e. Use 6–10 recognisable words

7. **A neonate is seen to twitch. Relevant points in the history include—**
   a. The mother is a known heroin addict
   b. The father has glomerulonephritis
   c. Penicillin was given to the mother in the first trimester
   d. The child was being bottle fed
   e. The child was small-for-dates

8. **Advanced bone age is a feature of—**
   a. Hypothyroidism
   b. Social deprivation
   c. Congenital adrenal hyperplasia
   d. Familial short stature
   e. Administration of cortisone

Answers overleaf

5. a. True Due to haemolysis
    b. False The main defect in Dubin–Johnson is in excretion of conjugated bilirubin from the liver cell
    c. False Again the main increase is in conjugated bilirubin
    d. True Due to haemolysis
    e. True Various mechanisms including immaturity of liver enzymes are responsible

6. a. True In a scissor fashion initially
    b. False Competence using a cup is acquired at about 18 months
    c. True
    d. False Response to commands is acquired by 12 months
    e. False Deliberate vocalisation is only beginning at this stage

7. a. True An opiate withdrawal syndrome may be seen in the infant
    b. False
    c. False Penicillin is one of the safest antibiotics for use in pregnancy
    d. True Some preparations contain too much phosphate, and hypocalcaemia results
    e. True Hypoglycaemia is common in small-for-dates infants

8. a. False It is characteristically retarded
    b. False Bone age may be moderately retarded
    c. True Initially these children may be tall for their age, but ultimately dwarfism occurs since the epiphyses fuse early
    d. False Bone age is normal
    e. False Short stature is due mainly to the inhibition of protein anabolism. Bone age may be a little retarded

9. **Characteristic non-articular features of Still's disease include—**
   a. Conjunctivitis
   b. Fleeting rash
   c. Leucocytosis
   d. Splenomegaly
   e. Rheumatoid nodules

10. **Characteristic features of acute lymphoblastic leukaemia include—**
    a. Tumour cells which react with antisera raised against B lymphocytes
    b. Better prognosis when the white cell count at presentation is very high
    c. Massive splenomegaly
    d. Disseminated intravascular coagulation
    e. Spread to the meninges unless prophylactic treatment to the central nervous system is given

11. **Characteristic features of phenylketonuria include—**
    a. Normal on physical examination at birth
    b. Eczema
    c. Tendency to venous thrombosis
    d. Cataracts
    e. Fair hair

12. **Characteristic features of Henoch–Schönlein purpura include—**
    a. Arthritis
    b. Membranous glomerulonephritis
    c. Rash involving the face
    d. Reduced serum complement
    e. Prolonged bleeding time

13. **Transplacental transfer of blood constituents may cause neonatal disease, when the mother is suffering from—**
    a. Hyperparathyroidism
    b. Tuberous sclerosis
    c. Idiopathic thrombocytopenic purpura
    d. Rheumatoid arthritis
    e. Biliary cirrhosis

Answers overleaf

9. a. False Iridocyclitis is characteristic
    b. True The rash may come and go within hours
    c. True Occasionally a leukaemoid reaction is seen
    d. True
    e. False Overall only about 10% have a positive rheumatoid factor and are likely to have nodules. These cases are mostly the subgroup where the disease starts at an older age

10. a. False Cells are usually of the null type and will not react with antisera to T or B cells
    b. False Although the initial response may be good, ultimately this group will have a poorer prognosis
    c. False Splenomegaly is mild to moderate in acute leukaemias
    d. False This is particularly associated with acute promyelocytic leukaemia
    e. True Before such prophylactic treatment, meningeal involvement often occurred even while otherwise the patient appeared to be in remission

11. a. True Hence the value of biochemical screening
    b. True
    c. False This is a feature of homocystinuria
    d. False
    e. True

12. a. True
    b. False The glomerulonephritis is usually focal
    c. False Buttocks and extensor surfaces are most commonly involved. The face can be involved in younger children
    d. False
    e. False The platelet count is normal

13. a. True Transient hypocalcaemia may result
    b. False The disorder is inherited by an autosomal dominant gene
    c. True Antiplatelet antibodies pass across the placenta
    d. False
    e. False

14. **Causes of liver cirrhosis in childhood include—**
    a. α_1-antitrypsin deficiency
    b. Coeliac disease
    c. Phenylketonuria
    d. Cow's milk intolerance
    e. Wilson's disease

15. **Characteristic presentations of cystic fibrosis include—**
    a. Abdominal distension at birth
    b. Rectal prolapse
    c. Asthma
    d. Diabetic ketoacidosis
    e. Iron deficiency anaemia

16. **In a boy of 4 with congenital adrenal hyperplasia—**
    a. The testes are enlarged
    b. Plasma ACTH levels are low
    c. Height is above normal
    d. Adrenalectomy is the treatment of choice
    e. A deficiency of 21-hydroxylase is most often the cause

17. **An infant is born at full term but weighs less than 2·5 kg. Complications which are characteristically associated include—**
    a. Meconium aspiration syndrome
    b. Intraventricular haemorrhage
    c. Hypoglycaemia
    d. Poor feeding
    e. Pulmonary haemorrhage

Answers overleaf

14. a. True It also causes neonatal hepatitis
    b. False
    c. False Though other disturbances of amino-acid handling may cause cirrhosis, e.g. tyrosinosis, cystinosis
    d. False
    e. True All cases of cirrhosis in childhood should be screened for this

15. a. True For obstruction (so-called 'meconium ileus') is present antenatally so that distension may be present from birth
    b. True
    c. False Recurrent infection is the main problem
    d. False Diabetes may complicate long-standing cases, but even then keto-acidosis is not common
    e. False Like other causes of pancreatic malabsorption, iron absorption is not seriously affected (blood loss from varices due to liver cirrhosis would tend to occur in established disease)

16. a. False They will be small. The excessive androgen comes from the adrenal, and testicular androgen production is suppressed
    b. False They are increased due to the feedback resulting from the enzyme block
    c. True Though dwarfism will ultimately occur because the epiphyses fuse early
    d. False Cortisone is used to suppress the increased ACTH drive which causes the excessive androgen production
    e. True

17. a. True
    b. False Certain complications tend to be common in the premature (as opposed to small-for-dates) infant and intraventricular haemorrhage is an example
    c. True
    d. False They usually feed greedily unless other complications prevent them
    e. True Particularly in association with hypothermia

18. **Muscular hypotonia without significant weakness is a characteristic feature of—**
    a. Cerebral palsy
    b. Rickets
    c. Down's syndrome
    d. Werdnig–Hoffmann disease (spinal muscular atrophy)
    e. Guillain–Barré syndrome

19. **Characteristic features of post-mature infants include—**
    a. Reduction in vernix
    b. Desquamating skin
    c. Absent scalp hair
    d. Meconium staining of the nails
    e. Alert appearance

20. **Failure of the anterior fontanelle to close by 18 months is a feature of—**
    a. Rickets
    b. Phenylketonuria
    c. Hydrocephalus
    d. Hypothyroidism
    e. Down's syndrome

Answers overleaf

18. a. False Spasticity is usual. Hypotonia is also seen, but would be associated with weakness
    b. True
    c. True
    d. False Weakness is prominent
    e. False

19. a. True Lanugo hair is also reduced
    b. True Both the reduction in vernix caseosa and desquamating skin are seen in the small-for-dates infant
    c. False It is increased
    d. True
    e. True

20. a. True
    b. False
    c. True The fontanelles become greatly enlarged and tense
    d. True Bone age is generally retarded
    e. False

Pathology

1. **Amyloid—**
   a. In multiple myeloma has a structure resembling immuno-globulin light chains
   b. Has a great affinity for Congo red
   c. In familial Mediterranean fever rarely involves the kidney
   d. Is seen in follicular carcinomas of the thyroid
   e. In primary amyloidosis characteristically involves small blood vessels

2. **Granuloma formation in the liver is a recognised feature of—**
   a. Chronic active hepatitis
   b. Brucellosis
   c. Berylliosis
   d. Hodgkin's disease
   e. Leptospirosis

3. **Haematological malignancies in which the cells are characteristically of B lymphocyte origin include—**
   a. Chronic lymphatic leukaemia
   b. Mycosis fungoides
   c. Myeloma
   d. Burkitt's lymphoma
   e. Acute lymphoblastic leukaemia

4. **Features more suggestive of Crohn's colitis than ulcerative colitis include—**
   a. Granuloma formation
   b. Pseudopolyp formation
   c. Crypt abscesses
   d. Sparing of the rectum
   e. Attachment of affected bowel to adjacent viscera

Answers overleaf

1. a. True Patients with other causes of 'primary' amyloidosis may also have paraprotein peaks
   b. True The basis of a diagnostic test
   c. False In this disease, the distribution follows that of secondary amyloid, and renal amyloid is common
   d. False It is seen in the medullary type of tumour
   e. True

2. a. False
   b. True As can other infections including tuberculosis, histoplasmosis and occasionally glandular fever
   c. True Due to industrial exposure. Sarcoidosis has several features in common including the presence of liver granulomas
   d. True Jaundice may be due to liver involvement, but also due to auto-immune haemolysis
   e. False

3. a. True A small number are T cell types, and they have a worse prognosis
   b. False T cell origin
   c. True
   d. True
   e. False Usually the cells have neither T nor B cell characteristics. The B cell variant has a worse prognosis

4. a. True But they may be absent
   b. False Typical of ulcerative colitis. Pseudopolyps are islands of mucosa left by denudation of the surrounding mucosa
   c. False Again typical of ulcerative colitis
   d. True The rectum is always involved in ulcerative colitis
   e. True This may lead to fistula formation

5. **Characteristic features of the liver in primary biliary cirrhosis include—**
   a. Green colour on naked-eye inspection
   b. Granuloma formation in the early stages
   c. Polymorph infiltration around the bile ducts
   d. Elevated copper levels
   e. Massive liver cell necrosis in the end stages

Answers overleaf

5. a. True
   b. True They are often absent in the later stages
   c. False Lymphocytes predominate
   d. True
   e. False By the end stages scarring and regenerating cirrhotic
             nodules predominate

Pharmacology

1. A fixed drug eruption is a characteristic unwanted effect of—
   a. Quinine
   b. Ampicillin
   c. Dapsone
   d. Phenolphthalein
   e. Chlorpromazine

2. Advantages of ACTH over prednisone include a lower incidence of—
   a. Osteoporosis
   b. Fluid retention
   c. Acne
   d. Adrenal insufficiency with intercurrent stress
   e. Growth retardation in children

3. In the treatment of acute intermittent porphyria drugs that may be safely used include—
   a. Methyl dopa for hypertension
   b. Diazepam for sedation
   c. Phenytoin for control of fits
   d. Pethidine for pain relief
   e. Sulphonamide for coincidental infection

4. Photosensitivity is a characteristic unwanted effect of—
   a. Tetracyclines
   b. Propranolol
   c. Chlorpropamide
   d. Carbenoxolone
   e. Chlorthiazide

5. Proximal myopathy is a characteristic unwanted effect of—
   a. Digoxin
   b. Clofibrate
   c. Neostigmine
   d. Chloroquine
   e. Bethanidine

Answers overleaf

1.   a.   True   A fixed eruption is one which recurs at the same site with repeated exposure
     b.   False
     c.   True
     d.   True   Barbiturates and sulphonamides are the other common causes
     e.   False   Photosensitivity is characteristic

2.   a.   True   ACTH causes release of anabolic as well as catabolic steroids
     b.   False
     c.   False   ACTH causes androgen release
     d.   True   The adrenals are not suppressed as is the case with prednisone
     e.   True   Again because ACTH has less catabolic effect

3.   a.   False   Methyl dopa may precipitate an attack. Propranolol is a better choice
     b.   True
     c.   False   Many anti-epileptics including barbiturates and other hydantoins precipitate intermittent porphyria
     d.   True
     e.   False

4.   a.   True   One of the commonest drug causes
     b.   False
     c.   True   The related sulphonamides are also a cause
     d.   False
     e.   True   Nalidixic acid and griseofulvin are other causes

5.   a.   False
     b.   True   Is only seen at high doses or in the presence of renal failure
     c.   False
     d.   True   Corticosteroids are probably the commonest cause
     e.   False

6. **Drugs that are metabolised by acetylation in the liver include—**
   a. Phenytoin
   b. Hydralazine
   c. Dapsone
   d. Tolbutamide
   e. Isoniazid

7. **Drugs that characteristically cause skin pigmentation as an unwanted effect include—**
   a. Chlorpromazine
   b. Phenylbutazone
   c. Chloroquine
   d. Streptomycin
   e. Busulphan

8. **Pulmonary fibrosis is a recognised unwanted effect of—**
   a. Hexamethonium
   b. Bleomycin
   c. Colchicine
   d. Phenytoin
   e. Nitrofurantoin

9. **Decreased efficiency of the contraceptive pill is recognised with the use of—**
   a. Rifampicin
   b. Warfarin
   c. Phenytoin
   d. Frusemide
   e. Hydralazine

10. **Glomerular damage is characteristic of the renal toxicity due to—**
    a. Penicillamine
    b. Cephaloridine
    c. Methysergide
    d. Troxidone
    e. Amphotericin B

Answers overleaf

6. a. False It is hydroxylated in the liver
   b. True Slow acetylators are more likely to get lupus erythematosus
   c. True
   d. False It is oxidised in the liver
   e. True Slow acetylators are more likely to get peripheral neuropathy

7. a. True
   b. False
   c. True Pigmentation is common. Pigmentation of the nail beds, bleaching of the hair, and retinal changes are also seen
   d. False
   e. True Pigmentation associated with weakness may simulate Addison's disease

8. a. True As with other little used ganglion blockers
   b. True As with some other cytotoxic agents, e.g. busulphan
   c. False
   d. False It may cause hilar lymphadenopathy
   e. True

9. a. True Due to hepatic enzyme induction
   b. False However, increased warfarin may be required for adequate anticoagulation
   c. True The effect, which is also noted with phenobarbitone is probably due to enzyme induction
   d. False
   e. False Though perhaps a hypertensive patient should not be taking the pill

10. a. True
    b. False Renal tubular damage is typical
    c. False The ureters are involved in retroperitoneal fibrosis
    d. True
    e. False Causes tubular damage including renal tubular acidosis

11. **Drugs that for the most part are excreted unchanged in the urine include —**
    a. Streptomycin
    b. Tetracycline
    c. Rifampicin
    d. Chloramphenicol
    e. Benzyl penicillin

12. **A predominantly cholestatic jaundice may complicate the use of —**
    a. Paracetamol
    b. Methyl testosterone
    c. Methyl dopa
    d. Chlorpropamide
    e. Primaquine

13. **Heparin —**
    a. Is a protein
    b. Is contained in mast cells
    c. Has a plasma half-life of about 8 hours
    d. Therapy can be monitored using the activated partial thromboplastin time
    e. Causes thrombocytopenia

14. **Disopyramide —**
    a. Is a myocardial depressant
    b. Should not be given if the patient is already on digoxin
    c. Is effective in controlling both atrial and ventricular arrhythmias
    d. May induce Parkinsonism
    e. Causes urinary retention

15. **Theophylline —**
    a. Is a major constituent of coffee
    b. Has a positive inotropic effect on the heart
    c. Is largely excreted unchanged by the kidneys
    d. Causes fits at toxic levels
    e. Needs to be given in higher doses to smokers

Answers overleaf

11. a. True
      b. True
      c. False It is metabolised in the liver
      d. False It is conjugated to the glucuronide in the liver
      e. True

12. a. False Hepatocellular damage follows overdosage
      b. True This causes a dose-related cholestasis, in common with oestrogens and anabolic steroids
      c. False
      d. True Due to a hypersensitivity reaction similar to that with chlorpromazine
      e. False Haemolysis in association with glucose-6-phosphate dehydrogenase deficiency is the usual mechanism of jaundice

13. a. False It is a mucopolysaccharide
      b. True
      c. False It is about 2 hours
      d. True
      e. True Thrombocytopenia due to platelet destruction is a recognised side effect

14. a. True Like many anti-arrhythmic agents
      b. False
      c. True
      d. False
      e. True Due to its anticholinergic effect

15. a. False It is contained in tea
      b. True
      c. False Only 7% is excreted unchanged
      d. True
      e. True Hepatic enzymes are induced in smokers

16. **Parkinsonism is an unwanted effect of—**
    a. Reserpine
    b. Chlorpromazine
    c. Bromocriptine
    d. Neostigmine
    e. Metoclopramide

17. **Drugs that cause systemic lupus erythematosus include—**
    a. Procainamide
    b. Gold
    c. Phenytoin
    d. Methotrexate
    e. Isoniazid

18. **Bromocriptine—**
    a. Is a dopamine antagonist
    b. Is used in the treatment of prolactinomas
    c. Occurs naturally in man
    d. Causes hypertension
    e. Suppresses lactation

19. **Hirsutism is a recognised side effect of—**
    a. Spironolactone
    b. Phenytoin
    c. Minoxidil
    d. Digoxin
    e. Clomiphene

20. **Harmful interactions are likely with the use of—**
    a. Alcohol and metronidazole
    b. Digoxin and nitrazepam
    c. Warfarin and propranolol
    d. Tolbutamide and phenylbutazone
    e. Rifampicin and para-aminosalicylic acid

Answers overleaf

16.
  a. True It causes depletion of dopamine at nerve endings
  b. True It is a dopamine receptor blocker
  c. False It is a dopamine agonist
  d. False It is an anticholinesterase
  e. True It probably works in the same way as chlorpromazine

17.
  a. True One of the commonest causes along with hydrallazine and phenytoin
  b. False
  c. True As can other anticonvulsants including primidone and ethosuximide
  d. False
  e. True

18.
  a. False It is a dopamine agonist
  b. True
  c. False It is a semi-synthetic ergot alkaloid
  d. False It is hypotensive
  e. True

19.
  a. False It causes gynaecomastia
  b. True
  c. True It occurs in most patients using this drug
  d. False
  e. False Hair loss has been reported

20.
  a. True Metronidazole inhibits aldehyde dehydrogenase and causes a disulfiram-like reaction
  b. False
  c. False
  d. True Both are highly protein bound. Dangerous hypoglycaemia may result
  e. True The absorption of rifampicin is reduced

21. **Metronidazole is effective against —**
    a. Actinomyces
    b. *Bacteroides fragilis*
    c. *Staphylococcus aureus*
    d. *Amoeba entahistolytica*
    e. *Clostridium welchii*

22. **Morphine —**
    a. Is conjugated in the liver
    b. Relaxes the gastro-oesophageal sphincter
    c. Causes pin-point pupils unresponsive to atropine
    d. May increase pressure in the biliary tree
    e. Causes urinary retention

23. **Drugs that are highly bound to plasma proteins (90% or greater) include —**
    a. Cloxacillin
    b. Gentamicin
    c. Phenylbutazone
    d. Chlorpromazine
    e. Digoxin

24. **Drugs with plasma half-lives of less than 12 hours include —**
    a. Phenylbutazone
    b. Phenobarbitone
    c. Tolbutamide
    d. Ethosuximide
    e. Propranolol

25. **Penicillamine —**
    a. Is contra-indicated in Still's disease
    b. May be safely restarted in some patients, once the platelet count has returned to normal, following an episode of thrombocytopenia
    c. Causes a reduction in the level of rheumatoid factor
    d. Is reserved for patients who have not responded to conventional therapy including a trial of steroids
    e. Absorption is reduced when iron is given concurrently

Answers overleaf

21. a. False The exception to the rule that it is effective against anaerobes
     b. True
     c. False
     d. True   It is also effective against *Giardia* and *Trichomonas*
     e. True

22. a. True
     b. False In the gastro-intestinal tract generally tone is increased while propulsive peristalsis is reduced
     c. False Atropine dilates the pupils
     d. True
     e. True   By increasing sphincter tone, and by acting centrally to alter attention to bladder stimuli

23. a. True   Unlike other penicillins
     b. False Negligible amounts are protein bound
     c. True   An important source of drug interaction
     d. True
     e. False

24. a. False 72 hours
     b. False 80 hours
     c. True   5 hours. There is less risk of hypoglycaemia than with chlorpropamide
     d. False Many anti-epileptic agents have long half-lives and can be given once daily
     e. True   3 hours

25. a. False It has been successfully used with the usual precautions
     b. True   Restart with a lower dose and increase slowly
     c. True
     d. False Especially in the younger patient it may be worth using early and certainly before steroids
     e. True   Iron is chelated in the gut and the complexes are not absorbed

Physiology

1. **Characteristic effects of excessive noradrenaline include—**
   a. Increased total peripheral resistance
   b. Fall in diastolic blood pressure
   c. Less effect than adrenaline on bronchial smooth muscle
   d. Relaxation of anal and bladder sphincters
   e. Inhibition of muscle contraction in the pregnant uterus

2. **Factors that increase the oxygen content of blood at a Po_2 of 50 mmHg (5·3 kPa) include an increase in—**
   a. pH
   b. Temperature
   c. Partial pressure of carbon dioxide
   d. 2, 3-diphosphoglycerate
   e. Haemoglobin

3. **In the proximal convoluted tubule—**
   a. About half the filtered uric acid is reabsorbed
   b. About 80 per cent of filtered water is reabsorbed under the influence of aldosterone
   c. Renin is produced
   d. Para-amino-hippuric acid is actively reabsorbed
   e. Potassium is reabsorbed

4. **Gastric acid release is increased by—**
   a. Hypoglycaemia
   b. Presence of food in the mouth
   c. Vaso-active intestinal peptide
   d. Acid in the duodenum
   e. Cholecystokinin-pancreozymin

5. **Cortisol—**
   a. Is essential for life
   b. Is required for excretion of a water load
   c. Release is mainly controlled by volume receptors in the great veins
   d. In excess gives pigmentation of the skin
   e. Has a plasma half-life of about 12 hours

Answers overleaf

1. a. True   Due to its α effects
   b. False   This is the case with β stimulation where the overall peripheral resistance is reduced
   c. True   Bronchodilation is a β effect
   d. False   Both are constricted
   e. False   This is a β effect and provides the rationale for the use of β stimulators in preventing premature labour

2. a. True   This shifts the oxygen dissociation curve to the left
   b. False   This shifts the oxygen dissociation curve to the right
   c. False   This also shifts the curve to the right
   d. False   Again the curve is to the right. Hypoxia and acidosis tend to increase the levels of 2, 3-diphosphoglycerate
   e. True

3. a. False   It is nearly all reabsorbed. Some is secreted in the distal convoluted tubule
   b. False   This water is absorbed irrespective of the action of aldosterone
   c. False   It is produced in the juxtaglomerular apparatus
   d. False   None is reabsorbed. Active secretion occurs in the distal tubule and its clearance gives an estimate of renal blood flow
   e. True

4. a. True   Via a vagal reflex
   b. True   Again via the vagus
   c. False   The reverse is true
   d. False
   e. False

5. a. True
   b. True   The water load test was commonly and sometimes dangerously used to diagnose Addison's disease
   c. False   ACTH release from the pituitary is the main factor and volume receptors have only a minor role in stimulating ACTH release
   d. False   This is an ACTH effect
   e. False   It is less than 2 hours

Psychiatry

1. **In phobic disorders—**
   a. Symptoms of anxiety are characteristic
   b. More males than females are affected
   c. Progressive disintegration of the personality occurs
   d. Prolonged exposure to the undesired situation is used in treatment
   e. ECT is the treatment of choice

2. **Well marked physical dependence is seen with—**
   a. Phenobarbitone
   b. Cannabis
   c. Cocaine
   d. Diamorphine
   e. Lysergic acid diethylamide (LSD)

3. **Characteristic features of anorexia nervosa include—**
   a. Hyperprolactinaemia
   b. Low FSH
   c. Low cholesterol
   d. Low growth hormone
   e. Hypokalaemia

4. **Factors that are associated with the development of anorexia nervosa include—**
   a. Delinquent behaviour in childhood
   b. Being female
   c. Family history of schizophrenia
   d. Thyroid dysfunction
   e. Large family size

5. **Characteristic features of childhood autism include—**
   a. Close relationship to parents
   b. Preoccupation with stereotyped routines
   c. Onset before the age of 5
   d. Accentuated ability in non-verbal communication
   e. Family history of schizophrenia

Answers overleaf

1. a. True
   b. False Many phobias, e.g. agoraphobia, are more common in women
   c. False
   d. True This is called 'flooding'. Desensitisation by gradual introduction of the unpleasant situation is also used
   e. False

2. a. True The withdrawal syndrome may include fits
   b. False
   c. False Physical dependence, if it occurs, is slight
   d. True
   e. False

3. a. False
   b. True LH is also low
   c. False It is often increased
   d. False It is often increased as in any state of under-nutrition
   e. True

4. a. False They are often excessively good
   b. True
   c. False
   d. False Various hormonal causes have been postulated but none proved. Bradycardia and low basal metabolic rate are a response to undernutrition and do not represent hypothyroidism
   e. False

5. a. False Failure to form close emotional relationships is typical
   b. True
   c. True It is rare after this age
   d. False Both verbal and non-verbal communication are impaired
   e. False The idea that autism is a type of schizophrenia is out of fashion

6. **Mutism is a recognised feature of—**
   a. Alcohol withdrawal
   b. Conversion hysteria
   c. Catatonic schizophrenia
   d. Depression
   e. Ganser states

7. **Depression is an unwanted effect of—**
   a. Cocaine
   b. Methyl dopa
   c. Nitrazepam
   d. Contraceptive pill
   e. Hydrallazine

8. **Characteristic features of obsessional states include—**
   a. Family history of schizophrenia
   b. Perseveration
   c. Onset in old age
   d. Good insight
   e. History of amphetamine abuse

9. **Disorientation in time is a characteristic feature of—**
   a. Korsakoff's psychosis
   b. Acute schizophrenic breakdown
   c. Hypomania
   d. Depressive psychosis
   e. Agoraphobia

10. **Echolalia is a recognised feature of—**
    a. Catatonic schizophrenia
    b. Anorexia nervosa
    c. Alzheimer's disease
    d. Childhood autism
    e. Petit mal epilepsy

Answers overleaf

6. a. False
     b. True
     c. True
     d. True In profound depressive stupor
     e. False This is a very rare condition, which may be a manifestation of hysteria. Approximate answers to questions are characteristic

7. a. False Cocaine is a stimulant. Excess may produce a toxic psychosis
     b. True Probably by causing depletion of neurotransmitters
     c. False
     d. True
     e. False Its effect is not mediated by monoamine neurotransmitter depletion

8. a. False Although schizophrenics may have obsessions, they are a minority of those with obsessional disorders
     b. False This is a feature of dementia
     c. False Onset may be at any age but more often in the young
     d. True They are usually all too aware of the problem
     e. False Amphetamine abuse can produce a psychosis

9. a. True Short-term memory loss with confabulation is typical
     b. False
     c. False
     d. False
     e. False

10. a. True A characteristic finding
     b. False
     c. True
     d. True Repetition of mannerisms and activities may also be seen
     e. False

11. Characteristic features of schizophrenia include—
    a. Obsessional thoughts
    b. Progression to dementia
    c. Depersonalisation
    d. Early morning wakening
    e. Thought withdrawal

12. Behaviour modification therapy is of use in—
    a. Paedophilia
    b. Schizophrenia
    c. Obsessional states
    d. Mania
    e. Agoraphobia

13. In a patient with an acute schizophrenic breakdown a bad ultimate prognosis is suggested by—
    a. Above-average intelligence
    b. Flattening of affect
    c. Sudden onset
    d. Normal premorbid personality
    e. Marked thought disorder

14. Risk factors for suicide include—
    a. Being married
    b. Age under 20 years
    c. Alcoholism
    d. A history of having discussed suicide with a friend
    e. Severe painful physical illness

15. Severe mental subnormality is characteristic of—
    a. Klinefelter's syndrome
    b. Lesch—Nyhan syndrome
    c. Neurofibromatosis
    d. Trisomy D
    e. Hurler's syndrome

Answers overleaf

11. a. False They are sometimes seen, but are not characteristic
     b. False
     c. True   This means a feeling of altered reality of self
     d. False A characteristic feature of depression
     e. True   A typical feature of schizophrenic thought disorder

12. a. True   Extensive use of behaviour modification is made in treating various sexual problems
     b. False
     c. True   The environment can be gradually altered so that it is not possible for the obsessional act to be carried out
     d. False
     e. True   Perhaps the main use is in phobic disorders

13. a. False The reverse is the case
     b. True
     c. False This suggests a precipitating factor and, if this is removed, the patient may not relapse
     d. False
     e. True

14. a. False The incidence is much higher in single, divorced or separated individuals
     b. False Though attempted suicides are common
     c. True
     d. True
     e. True

15. a. False Mild retardation is quite common
     b. True   A disorder of uric acid metabolism. The tendency to self-mutilation is particularly characteristic and distressing
     c. False
     d. True   Cardiac abnormalities and cleft palate are also characteristic
     e. True

16. **Characteristic features of morphine withdrawal include —**

    a. Excessive yawning
    b. Hypotension
    c. Muscle cramps
    d. Dry eyes
    e. Diarrhoea

17. **In tardive dyskinesia —**

    a. There is usually a history of having recently started phenothiazines
    b. Intramuscular benztropine is rapidly effective in reversing the changes
    c. Facial grimacing is characteristic
    d. Intention tremor is a recognised sign
    e. Reduction in the dosage of phenothiazines may precipitate an attack

18. **Grandiose delusions are a recognised feature of —**

    a. Schizophrenia
    b. Frontal lobe tumour
    c. Mania
    d. Obsessional neurosis
    e. Amphetamine intoxication

19. **Characteristic features of acute mania include —**

    a. Retention of insight
    b. Flight of ideas
    c. Confabulation
    d. Distractability
    e. Family history of depression

20. **Recognised features of depression include —**

    a. Poor concentration
    b. Delusional perceptions
    c. Hypochondriasis
    d. Delusions of bodily influence
    e. Weight loss

Answers overleaf

16. a. True One of the early features
    b. False Moderate hypertension is often seen
    c. True
    d. False Running eyes and rhinorrhoea are usual
    e. True

17. a. False It is usually seen in patients on long-term phenothiazines
    b. False Treatment is difficult. Prevention by 'drug holidays' has been suggested, where phenothiazines are stopped at regular intervals
    c. True
    d. False This is a sign of cerebellar disease
    e. True

18. a. True Though schizophrenia is not a common cause
    b. True
    c. True
    d. False
    e. True Any other causes of acute confusional states could also be responsible

19. a. False It is lost
    b. True
    c. False This is making up answers to cover a memory defect. It is characteristic of Korsakoff's psychosis
    d. True They notice many things and can be easily set off on a different line of thought
    e. True In bipolar illness (alternating mania and depression) a family history is especially common

20. a. True Mental processes are slowed though accuracy is usually preserved
    b. False Delusions in depression are secondary to the affective state
    c. True
    d. False A characteristic feature of schizophrenia
    e. True

Poisoning

1. **Characteristic early features of salicylate poisoning in an adult include—**
   a. Coma
   b. Acidosis
   c. Tinnitus
   d. Renal failure
   e. Sweating

2. **Recognised features of barbiturate poisoning include—**
   a. Liver necrosis
   b. Hypotension
   c. Hypothermia
   d. Bullous rash
   e. Reversal of respiratory depression by naloxone

3. **In acute iron poisoning—**
   a. Delay in the onset of symptoms is recognised
   b. Stricture of the stomach occurs as a late complication
   c. Desferrioxamine acts so slowly that it is of little use
   d. A history of paint spraying may be obtained
   e. Liver necrosis is a recognised complication

4. **In acute paracetamol poisoning—**
   a. Loss of consciousness is characteristic
   b. Those on long term barbiturates are less severely affected
   c. Acute tubular necrosis is a recognised complication
   d. There is little risk if the patient survives the first 24 hours
   e. Administration of penicillamine may prevent liver necrosis

Answers overleaf

1. a. False The patient is often awake and agitated. Coma tends to be late and serious
   b. False Early on, alkalosis resulting from hyperventilation is the rule. Acidosis occurs later. In children acidosis may be present at an earlier stage
   c. True   Often one of the first signs of overdosage
   d. False An occasional late complication
   e. True

2. a. False
   b. True   Due to a direct toxic effect on the myocardium as well as decreased venous return to the heart because of peripheral venous pooling
   c. True
   d. True   Glutethimide and tricyclic overdosage also cause bullous rashes
   e. False Naloxone is used in opiate overdosage

3. a. True   Some hours may elapse
   b. True
   c. False Given directly into the stomach and also parenterally it chelates and removes useful amounts of iron
   d. False This would be a possibility in lead poisoning
   e. True   And may be fatal

4. a. False It is uncommon unless other sedative drugs have also been taken
   b. False Paracetamol is converted to a toxic metabolite in the liver, and this process will be increased if liver enzymes are already induced by barbiturates
   c. True   Though liver necrosis is more common
   d. False Liver necrosis may only become apparent after 48 hours
   e. False Cysteamine, or more recently *N*-acetylcysteamine, has been used successfully

5. **Characteristic features of severe poisoning by the European Adder (Vipera berus) include—**
   a. Severe hypotension
   b. Absence of local reaction to the snake bite
   c. Neurotoxicity
   d. Neutrophil leucocytosis
   e. Abdominal pain

Answers overleaf

5. a. True   This is a feature of severe poisoning but may also result from a vasovagal attack
   b. False   This can generally be taken to indicate that no poisoning has occurred
   c. False   This is a feature of bites with elapids (cobras) and sea snakes
   d. True
   e. True

Renal Diseases

1. **Features in the nephrotic syndrome indicating a bad ultimate prognosis include—**
   a. Hyperlipidaemia
   b. Highly selective proteinuria
   c. Glomerular filtration rate of 10 ml per minute
   d. Proteinuria of greater than 10 g in 24 hours
   e. Onset in childhood

2. **Causes of renal papillary necrosis include—**
   a. Amyloidosis
   b. Phenacetin
   c. Sickle cell disease
   d. Renal tubular acidosis
   e. Diabetes mellitus

3. **A reduced serum complement level is characteristic of—**
   a. Minimal lesion glomerulonephritis
   b. Lupus nephritis
   c. Membranous glomerulonephritis
   d. Acute post-streptococcal glomerulonephritis
   e. Membrano-proliferative glomerulonephritis

4. **Causes of hypokalaemia include—**
   a. Addison's disease
   b. Carbenoxolone
   c. Chronic pyelonephritis
   d. Fresh water drowning
   e. Bronchial carcinoma

Answers overleaf

1.   a.   False   This is generally of no prognostic significance. Nephrotic syndrome due to systemic lupus is said not to give hyperlipidaemia
     b.   False
     c.   True   If renal failure of this degree has developed the outlook would generally be poor
     d.   False
     e.   False   Minimal lesion glomerulonephritis with a relatively good prognosis is common in childhood

2.   a.   False
     b.   True   The classic cause of papillary necrosis
     c.   True   Ischaemia is caused by sludging of red cells in the renal papillae
     d.   False
     e.   True   May present chronically as is usual with other causes of papillary necrosis, or sometimes acutely in association with severe infection

3.   a.   False
     b.   True
     c.   False   Though complement is deposited in the glomeruli in this and many other renal diseases, complement production often enables the serum level to remain normal
     d.   True
     e.   True   A profound hypocomplementaemia is usual

4.   a.   False   Hyperkalaemia is usual
     b.   True   Due to the aldosterone-like action
     c.   True   Potassium loss is occasionally marked
     d.   False   Haemolysis due to hypotonic fresh water causes hyperkalaemia
     e.   True   Due to ectopic ACTH production

5. **A patient has suffered considerable blood loss and has been oliguric for some hours. Factors that point towards acute tubular necrosis which will not be reversed by fluid replacement include an increase in—**

   a. Blood urea
   b. Urinary sodium excretion
   c. Urinary urea excretion
   d. Urinary osmolarity
   e. Urine volume

6. **A strongly acid urine is a recognised feature of—**

   a. Severe pyloric stenosis
   b. Renal tubular acidosis
   c. Chronic obstructive airways disease
   d. Chronic renal failure
   e. Urinary tract infection with *Proteus*

7. **Features that suggest the presence of underlying chronic renal failure in a patient with acute renal failure include—**

   a. Bilateral small kidneys on pyelography
   b. Renal osteodystrophy
   c. Reduced plasma bicarbonate
   d. Raised serum phosphate
   e. Normocytic normochromic anaemia

8. **An elevated blood urea is characteristic of—**

   a. Severe pyloric stenosis
   b. Nephrotic syndrome
   c. Excessive antidiuretic hormone secretion
   d. Liver failure
   e. Gastrointestinal haemorrhage

Answers overleaf

5. a. False   Any cause of extracellular fluid volume depletion will increase the blood urea
    b. True   In tubular necrosis sodium is not reabsorbed
    c. False   In tubular necrosis excretion of urea is reduced
    d. False   In tubular necrosis the osmolarity falls due to failure to concentrate urine, while in volume depletion the urine is keenly concentrated
    e. False   Oliguria should persist

6. a. True   The severe fluid depletion causes sodium reabsorption (with loss of hydrogen and potassium ions) to override acid-base considerations. Since potassium is already low hydrogen ion is lost at the distal tubule despite the systemic alkalosis
    b. False   Failure to produce an acid urine is the problem
    c. True   In an attempt to compensate for the respiratory acidosis
    d. True   Despite an overall reduction in hydrogen ion excretion and systemic acidosis. The mechanism of acid urine is obscure
    e. False   *Proteus* splits urea, resulting in production of ammonia

7. a. True   Small kidneys are typical of chronic glomerulo-nephritis and chronic pyelonephritis
    b. True
    c. False   Acidosis occurs in acute and chronic renal failure
    d. False   Again this occurs in both acute and chronic renal failure
    e. True   Anaemia takes time to develop in acute renal failure

8. a. True   Due to dehydration
    b. False   Renal failure is not necessarily a feature of nephrotic syndrome
    c. False   Haemodilution occurs
    d. False   Urea is low due to failure of liver synthesis
    e. True   Due to ingestion of a large amount of protein from breakdown of blood

9. **Characteristic features of the nephrotic syndrome include—**
   a. Increased plasma volume
   b. Hyperlipidaemia
   c. Reduced urinary sodium excretion
   d. Bence–Jones protein in the urine
   e. Leuconychia

10. **There is a characteristic association between high renin levels and—**
    a. Conn's syndrome
    b. Addison's disease
    c. Propranolol therapy
    d. Increased potassium intake
    e. Essential hypertension

11. **Causes of hyperchloraemic acidosis include—**
    a. Diabetic ketoacidosis
    b. Ureterosigmoidostomy
    c. Renal tubular acidosis
    d. Chronic obstructive airways disease
    e. Pyloric stenosis

12. **A clinical picture of fulminating acute nephritis occurs in—**
    a. Minimal lesion glomerulonephritis
    b. Polyarteritis nodosa
    c. Post-streptococcal glomerulonephritis
    d. Diabetes
    e. Membranous glomerulonephritis

Answers overleaf

9. a. False The intravascular volume is reduced due to loss of fluid from the hypoalbuminaemic circulation. This induces hyperaldosteronism and retention of fluid, which in turn is lost from the circulation to become tissue oedema
    b. True
    c. True Due to the secondary hyperaldosteronism
    d. False
    e. True As with other hypoalbuminaemic states

10. a. False Increased aldosterone is the primary event and this lowers renin by negative feed back
    b. True The low sodium and low renal perfusion pressure elevate renin
    c. False The sympathetic nervous system causes renin release
    d. False Renin levels are reduced
    e. False Generally renin is normal

11. a. False Various unmeasured anions constitute an 'anion gap'
    b. True Due to exchange of bicarbonate for chloride across the intestinal epithelium
    c. True Systemic acidosis is due to an inability to produce an acid urine. Chloride increases to fill the anion gap
    d. False A compensated respiratory acidosis is usual
    e. False

12. a. False It usually presents as nephrotic syndrome
    b. True Nephritis also occurs in other vasculitic disorders
    c. True The classic acute nephritis of children. The prognosis is usually good but some progress rapidly with fatal outcome
    d. False
    e. False Though it may present with haematuria, an acute fulminating course is not a feature

13. **In renal artery stenosis—**
    a. Surgery may help
    b. The affected kidney is small
    c. An intravenous pyelogram shows delay in the appearance of contrast
    d. Aldosterone levels are depressed
    e. Urine from the affected kidney is high in sodium

14. **Recognised features of renal tubular acidosis include—**
    a. Systemic alkalosis
    b. Hypokalaemia
    c. Repeated urinary tract infection
    d. Nephrocalcinosis
    e. Hypochloraemia

15. **A woman in end-stage renal failure who starts regular haemodialysis can confidently expect—**
    a. Anaemia to improve
    b. To avoid developing renal bone disease
    c. To observe no fluid restriction
    d. Nausea and vomiting to improve
    e. Return of fertility

Answers overleaf

13.   a.   True   But medical therapy is also effective in many cases
       b.   True
       c.   True   The disappearance of contrast is also delayed
       d.   False
       e.   False   It is low, as is the urine volume, due to increased reabsorption. Selective ureteric catheterisation to determine this is less used now

14.   a.   False   There is acidosis
       b.   True   Potassium is lost at the distal tubule instead of hydrogen ions, which cannot be excreted
       c.   True
       d.   True   Associated with hypercalciuria
       e.   False   Chloride is elevated to fill the anion gap left by low bicarbonate

15.   a.   False   Occasionally it does, but not usually. It may be worsened by leakage of blood, and further reduction in erythropoietin if bilateral nephrectomy is done
       b.   False   As patients do not die from uraemia, metabolic bone problems may become more apparent
       c.   False   After onset of dialysis urinary output may fall and fluid restriction must be observed if heart failure and hypertension are to be avoided
       d.   True   Where these are due to uraemia
       e.   False   While libido and periods may return, fertility rarely does

Respiratory Medicine

1. **Causes of massive haemoptysis include—**
   a. Bronchiectasis
   b. Tuberculosis
   c. Chronic bronchitis
   d. Bronchial carcinoma
   e. Systemic lupus erythematosus

2. **Causes of finger clubbing include—**
   a. Fibrosing alveolitis
   b. Chronic bronchitis
   c. Ulcerative colitis
   d. Bronchial adenoma
   e. Mesothelioma of the pleura

3. **Hypertrophic pulmonary osteoarthropathy is associated with—**
   a. Gynaecomastia
   b. Periosteal new bone formation
   c. Bronchial neoplasia, usually of oat cell type
   d. Alleviation by vagotomy
   e. Pleural mesothelioma

4. **A man of 60 has a bronchial neoplasm. Attempts at curative resection are contraindicated if he has—**
   a. Horner's syndrome
   b. Forced expiratory volume in one second of 3 litres
   c. Pleural effusion
   d. Sensori-motor neuropathy
   e. Left recurrent laryngeal nerve involvement

Answers overleaf

1. a. True   The quantity of haemoptysis is not a reliable guide to causation, but there are few causes of really massive haemoptysis
    b. True   A cavity may erode a branch of the pulmonary artery. Bleeding can be fatal
    c. False Haemoptysis if it occurs is slight and other causes should always be excluded
    d. True
    e. False Haemoptysis is a recognised feature but is usually slight

2. a. True
    b. False Some might dispute this, but 'false' is the required answer
    c. True   Other diseases such as Crohn's, malabsorption and liver cirrhosis also cause it
    d. False
    e. True

3. a. True   Probably due to gonadotrophin formation
    b. True   This can be seen on X-ray of wrists and ankles
    c. False Finger clubbing and hypertrophic pulmonary osteo-arthropathy are more often seen with squamous carcinomas
    d. True   Excision of the tumour or steroids may also help
    e. True

4. a. True   The sympathetic chain is involved and this implies local extension
    b. False This is an acceptable forced expiratory volume
    c. False The effusion may only be secondary to infection. If malignant cells are present spread to the pleura can be inferred
    d. False This is a non-metastatic manifestation
    e. True   This implies local extension

5. **Bronchial adenomas—**

   a. Occur more frequently in smokers
   b. Can usually be resected endoscopically
   c. May present with a lung abscess
   d. May give rise to lesions of the left side of the heart
   e. Can be locally invasive

6. **Sarcoidosis—**

   a. Is commonest in those over 50 years of age
   b. Should always be treated with steroids
   c. Presenting with erythema nodosum has a poor prognosis
   d. Characteristically gives a positive tuberculin test
   e. Usually responds to antituberculous therapy

7. **A boy of 18 has a moderately severe attack of asthma. One would expect to find—**

   a. Po_2 less than 60 mmHg (8.0 kPa)
   b. Pco_2 greater than 60 mmHg (8.0 kPa)
   c. Raised plasma bicarbonate
   d. Immediate relief by intravenous injection of hydrocortisone
   e. Dehydration

8. **An exacerbation of Farmer's lung—**

   a. Is commoner in summer
   b. Is characterised by intense wheeze
   c. Produces eosinophilia in the peripheral blood
   d. Is excluded by the absence of precipitating antibodies
   e. May respond to steroids

Answers overleaf

5. a. False
    b. False   Usually only the 'tip of the iceberg' can be seen through the bronchoscope
    c. True   By bronchial obstruction
    d. True   They produce 5-hydroxy-tryptophan, which is released into the pulmonary venous circulation and hence reaches the left side of the heart. With carcinoids from other sites the active peptides are broken down in the lungs
    e. True   Although this calls into question the term 'adenoma'

6. a. False
    b. False   Many cases resolve without steroids. Steroids are generally given for involvement of the eyes, the heart and the nervous system. Severe lung involvement is also an indication
    c. False   This presentation, often associated with bilateral hilar lymphadenopathy, usually clears without specific therapy
    d. False   Cell mediated immunity is depressed
    e. False   Such a response would suggest that tuberculosis was the correct diagnosis

7. a. True
    b. False   Generally carbon dioxide is adequately excreted. If retention occurs artificial ventilation should be considered
    c. False   In respiratory acidosis with carbon dioxide retention such a compensatory metabolic change occurs, for example in chronic bronchitis
    d. False   It takes a few hours
    e. True   It may need correction with intravenous fluids

8. a. False   It occurs when mouldy stored hay is used for winter feeding
    b. False   Airways obstruction is not a prominent feature
    c. False   This is characteristic of asthma
    d. False   These are not found in some typical cases
    e. True

9. **Mesothelioma of the pleura—**
   a. May follow asbestos exposure 30 years previously
   b. Characteristically develops on a pleural plaque
   c. Is a prescribed disease
   d. May produce a chest X-ray resembling a pleural effusion
   e. Is slowly progressive over many years following diagnosis

10. **Characteristic features of silicosis include—**
    a. Worsening of symptoms when returning to work after a few days off
    b. Predisposition to tuberculosis
    c. Exertional dyspnoea
    d. Response to steroids
    e. Focal fibrosis of the lower lobes

11. **Features of idiopathic pulmonary haemosiderosis include—**
    a. Recurrent haemoptysis
    b. Onset in those over 50 years of age
    c. Hypochromic anaemia
    d. Haemosiderin laden macrophages in the sputum
    e. Satisfactory response to desferrioxamine

12. **The following may be found in acute miliary tuberculosis—**
    a. Normal chest X-ray
    b. Negative tuberculin test
    c. Aplastic anaemia
    d. Occurrence in individuals who have had BCG
    e. Splenomegaly

13. **A single 3-cm rounded shadow outside the hilum on chest X-ray with no other abnormality could be due to—**
    a. Hydatid disease
    b. Secondary carcinoma
    c. Sarcoidosis
    d. Wegener's granulomatosis
    e. Pulmonary alveolar proteinosis

Answers overleaf

9. a. True   Such cases occur
    b. False No obvious relation to pleural plaques is recognised
    c. True   And compensation is available
    d. True
    e. False Despite treatment death is usually within two years

10. a. False This is characteristic of byssinosis
    b. True   This should always be suspected if a rapid deterioration occurs
    c. True
    d. False
    e. False The focal fibrosis tends to affect the upper lobes

11. a. True
    b. False It is commoner in young people
    c. True   Due to blood loss from haemoptysis
    d. True   Although characteristic they are by no means specific
    e. False Overall iron overload is not a problem

12. a. True   The tubercles may be too small to be seen
    b. True   Especially with overwhelming tuberculous infection the immune response may be depressed
    c. True   This usually recovers after antituberculous treatment
    d. False Acute miliary tuberculosis and tuberculous meningitis rarely if ever occur after BCG
    e. True

13. a. True
    b. True
    c. False Masses due to lymph nodes may occur in the hilum
    d. True
    e. False This rare disease is characterised by a diffuse infiltration of the alveoli with a lipoprotein

14. Asbestosis—
    a. Produces a restrictive lung defect
    b. Is functionally more severe when many asbestos bodies are found in the sputum
    c. In smokers protects against bronchial carcinoma
    d. Characteristically produces lung nodules
    e. Is usually severe if pleural plaques are seen on chest X-ray

15. In emphysema the following parameters of lung function are reduced—
    a. Ratio of forced expiratory volume in one second to forced vital capacity
    b. Residual volume
    c. Peak flow rate
    d. Lung compliance
    e. Transfer factor for carbon monoxide ($T_L CO$)

16. Characteristic findings on examination of pleural fluid include—
    a. A high sugar level in rheumatoid arthritis
    b. A protein concentration of 5 g/l in bronchial carcinoma
    c. Numerous polymorphs in tuberculosis
    d. Numerous red blood cells in pulmonary infarction
    e. Raised amylase in effusion following pancreatitis

17. A lateral chest X-ray reveals a mass posteriorly. This is characteristic of a—
    a. Thymoma
    b. Tuberculous abscess
    c. Pericardial cyst
    d. Bronchogenic cyst
    e. Neuroblastoma

Answers overleaf

14. a. True
b. False   Asbestos bodies only indicate exposure to asbestos, and do not by themselves indicate lung changes
c. False   The risk is compounded
d. False   Fibrotic changes are diffuse affecting especially the lower lobes
e. False   These do not indicate, or correlate with, changes in the lung parenchyma

15. a. True   Emphysema causes airways obstruction
b. False   It is increased due to air trapping
c. True   Again due to airways obstruction
d. False   There is loss of elastic tissue and therefore the lung volume will change more easily for a given pressure change
e. True   Although we think of transfer factor as a measure of diffusion being characteristically depressed in diseases affecting the alveolus (such as fibrosing alveolitis) it is also affected by ventilation/perfusion abnormalities. It is better to think of it as a measure of overall gas exchange and this is impaired in emphysema

16. a. False   The sugar level is low
b. False   Carcinomas usually result in an exudate—protein greater than 30 g/l
c. False   Numerous lymphocytes are characteristic
d. True   But also think of a malignant effusion
e. True

17. a. False   The thymus is sited anteriorly
b. True   These may arise in the vertebrae and track downwards
c. False   These cysts occur at the inferior cardiophrenic angles. Remember the heart is anterior in the mediastinum
d. False   These occur near major bronchi in the superior and anterior part of the mediastinum
e. True   As with other tumours of neurogenic origin such as neurofibromas and ganglioneuroblastomas

18. **Recognised findings in sarcoidosis include—**
    a. Bilateral facial nerve palsy
    b. Exfoliative dermatitis
    c. Erythema multiforme
    d. Heart block
    e. Lacrimal gland enlargement

19. **Causes of diffuse lung fibrosis include—**
    a. Byssinosis
    b. Rheumatoid arthritis
    c. Pneumococcal pneumonia
    d. Bleomycin
    e. Goodpasture's syndrome

20. **There is a recognised association between pneumothorax and—**
    a. Exposure to aluminium
    b. Acute pulmonary oedema
    c. Ehlers–Danlos syndrome
    d. Tuberculosis
    e. Pleural mesothelioma

Answers overleaf

18. a. True It may be part of Heerfordt's syndrome, which also includes parotitis and uveitis

b. False Skin findings in sarcoidosis include erythema nodosum, lupus pernio and a generalised papular or nodular eruption. Exfoliation is not a feature

c. False Erythema nodosum is the typical lesion

d. True Due to sarcoid granulomas affecting the conducting system

e. True

19. a. False In the chronic stages of byssinosis, bronchitis and emphysema occur but no fibrosis

b. True As with other connective tissue disorders

c. False

d. True As with a long list of other drugs

e. True Pulmonary haemorrhage occurs and lung fibrosis may ensue

20. a. True Pneumothorax is also seen in other occupational diseases, e.g. coal workers' pneumoconiosis, silicosis, berylliosis

b. False

c. True There is abnormal connective tissue. Small subpleural cysts result and these can rupture

d. True

e. False

Rheumatology

1. **Characteristic features of Reiter's disease include—**
   a. Cutaneous vasculitis
   b. Pericarditis
   c. Scleromalacia
   d. Sacroiliitis
   e. Eosinophilia

2. **Characteristic features of polymyalgia rheumatica include—**
   a. Raised creatinine phosphokinase
   b. Response to steroids within a few days
   c. Abnormal EMG
   d. Normocytic anaemia
   e. Morning stiffness

3. **Hyperuricaemia is found in—**
   a. Chronic myeloid leukaemia
   b. Hyperthyroidism
   c. Low dose salicylate administration
   d. Starvation
   e. Xanthinuria

4. **Mouth ulcers are a recognised feature of—**
   a. Psoriasis
   b. Hyperthyroidism
   c. Ulcerative colitis
   d. Reiter's disease
   e. Syphilis

5. **Features more characteristic of the drug-induced form of systemic lupus than other cases of systemic lupus include—**
   a. Equal sex incidence
   b. Kidney involvement
   c. Fatal outcome
   d. Low complement levels
   e. Antibodies to native double strand DNA

Answers overleaf

1. a. False This is characteristic of seropositive arthritis
   b. False Again a feature of seropositive arthritis
   c. False Conjunctivitis and iritis are the usual eye changes in Reiter's
   d. True As with all seronegative arthritis
   e. False

2. a. False Muscle enzymes are usually normal
   b. True Diagnostic in itself
   c. False
   d. True
   e. True

3. a. True As with many haematological and other malignancies
   b. False But it does occur in hypothyroidism
   c. True At higher doses proximal tubular reabsorption of urate is reduced
   d. True
   e. False Due to absence of xanthine oxidase, uric acid is not produced

4. a. False
   b. False
   c. True
   d. True Other causes include simple aphthous ulceration, trauma, coeliac disease and Behçet's disease
   e. True

5. a. True In other cases females are much more commonly affected
   b. False
   c. False Recovery after stopping the offending drug often occurs
   d. False
   e. False

6. **Characteristic features of systemic sclerosis include—**
   a. Long-term benefit of corticosteroids
   b. Raynaud's phenomenon
   c. Obstructive ventilatory defect
   d. Asymmetrical polyarthritis
   e. Telangiectasia

7. **Features of ankylosing spondylitis include—**
   a. Presentation with peripheral arthritis
   b. Apical lung fibrosis
   c. Osteophytes on X-ray of lumbar spine
   d. Aortic incompetence
   e. Amyloidosis

8. **Features recognised as normal in joint fluid include—**
   a. Low viscosity
   b. Cell count of 200 per mm^3 (0.2×10^9/l)
   c. Sugar level half that of blood
   d. Presence of fibrin clot
   e. A few crystals of hydroxyapatite

9. **Recognised skin manifestations of dermatomyositis include—**
   a. Squamous carcinoma of the skin
   b. Yellow nails
   c. Periorbital oedema
   d. Nail fold haemorrhages
   e. Xanthomas

10. **In a patient with symmetrical polyarthritis findings that would point towards a diagnosis of lupus erythematosus as opposed to rheumatoid arthritis include—**
    a. Positive Coombs' test
    b. Subperiosteal erosions
    c. A skin rash
    d. Subcutaneous nodules
    e. Psychosis

Answers overleaf

6. a. False No effect is proved
    b. True
    c. False A restrictive lung defect is usual
    d. False Symmetrical polyarthritis is usual
    e. True

7. a. True It may resemble rheumatoid arthritis
    b. True And is occasionally complicated by cavitation
    c. False Syndesmophytes are the typical finding
    d. True
    e. True

8. a. False It is normally high due to hyaluronic acid
    b. True
    c. False This would suggest septic or tuberculous arthritis
    d. False None should be present as normal fluid does not contain fibrinogen
    e. False Crystals are not normally present

9. a. False The association is with internal malignancy
    b. False Classically seen in the yellow nail syndrome, which is associated with lymphoedema
    c. True Associated with the typical heliotrope rash
    d. True
    e. False

10. a. True It is found in 15 per cent of patients with SLE. It is rare in rheumatoid arthritis
    b. False Erosive arthritis is less common in SLE
    c. True
    d. False Much more common in rheumatoid arthritis
    e. True A well recognised presentation of systemic lupus

11. Punched-out lesions on X-ray of the hands are recognised in—

    a.   Marfan's syndrome
    b.   Hypertrophic pulmonary osteoarthropathy
    c.   Gout
    d.   Sarcoid
    e.   Brucellosis

12. Joints involved more characteristically in rheumatoid arthritis than osteoarthritis include—

    a.   First carpometacarpal joint of the hand
    b.   Acromioclavicular joint
    c.   Temperomandibular joint
    d.   Wrists
    e.   Apophyseal joints of the lower cervical vertebrae

13. A polyarthropathy is a recognised feature of—

    a.   Acromegaly
    b.   Thyrotoxicosis
    c.   Sarcoidosis
    d.   Phaeochromocytoma
    e.   Syringomyelia

14. In a patient with psoriatic arthropathy characteristic features include—

    a.   Iritis
    b.   Involvement of the distal interphalangeal joints
    c.   Female preponderance
    d.   Pitting of the nails
    e.   Mononeuritis multiplex

Answers overleaf

11. a. False Arachnodactyly may be noticed
    b. False Periosteal new bone formation at the wrists and ankles is typical
    c. True
    d. True They do not usually cause symptoms but tend to be associated with skin sarcoid
    e. False Occasionally X-ray changes are seen in the spine

12. a. False This is typical of osteoarthritis
    b. False Again typical of osteoarthritis
    c. True
    d. True Not commonly affected in osteoarthritis unless as a sequel to injury
    e. False Rheumatoid arthritis tends to affect the upper cervical spine

13. a. True A symmetrical polyarthropathy may be seen
    b. False But occurs in myxoedema
    c. True An acute polyarthropathy may be seen with erythema nodosum, but a chronic form also occurs
    d. False As there are a great number of rare causes of polyarthropathy it can be hard to have courage and put 'false'
    e. False Other rarer causes of polyarthropathy to remember include haemochromatosis, hyperparathyroidism, hyperlipidaemia and many acute infections

14. a. False Although iritis is strongly associated with seronegative arthritis, if it occurs in psoriasis it is very rare
    b. True
    c. False The sex incidence is roughly equal
    d. True Psoriatic joint disease is nearly always associated with nail pitting
    e. False This is a feature of seropositive disease

15. **Features of polyarteritis nodosa include—**
    a. Focal glomerulonephritis
    b. Commoner in females
    c. Keratoderma blennorrhagia
    d. Myocardial infarction
    e. Abdominal pain

Answers overleaf

15. a. True
    b. False   Unlike the other collagen diseases it is commoner in males
    c. False   A feature of Reiter's disease. But there are a great many skin signs in polyarteritis
    d. True   The coronary arteries may be involved
    e. True   Abdominal complaints of various types are common

Sexually Transmitted Diseases

1. **Characteristic features of secondary syphilis include—**
   a. Mucosal erosions
   b. Painless lymphadenopathy
   c. Severe prostration
   d. Interstitial keratitis
   e. Itchy rash

2. **The fluorescent treponemal antibody test is characteristically positive—**
   a. In *Treponema pertenue* infection
   b. In glandular fever
   c. Within 3 weeks of infection with *Treponema pallidum*
   d. In tabes dorsalis
   e. In secondary syphilis

3. **Findings in tabes dorsalis include—**
   a. Generalised hypertonia
   b. Bilateral ptosis
   c. Pupils that react to light but not to accommodation
   d. Upgoing plantars
   e. Trophic ulcers

4. **Characteristic features of an acute attack of gonorrhoea include—**
   a. Incubation period of 2 weeks
   b. Diarrhoea
   c. Response to tetracycline
   d. Reliable diagnosis by serology
   e. Genital ulceration

5. **Lymphogranuloma venereum—**
   a. Is endemic throughout the United States
   b. May be complicated by urethral stricture
   c. Is characterised by massive penile ulceration
   d. Erythema nodosum is a recognised feature
   e. Is best treated with penicillin

Answers overleaf

1. a. True
   b. True
   c. False   The generalised illness is usually mild
   d. False   This is characteristic of congenital syphilis. Iritis is the main but uncommon eye complication of secondary syphilis
   e. False   The rash is non-irritant

2. a. True   Syphilitic serology does not distinguish between treponema pallidum and other treponemal strains
   b. False   Although a transient positive Wassermann occurs
   c. False   Although the test is the first to become positive, this is still too early
   d. True
   e. True   Serology should be positive by this stage

3. a. False   Hypotonia is typical
   b. True
   c. False   The other way about
   d. False   Tabes does not affect upper motor neurones
   e. True

4. a. False   It is 2–6 days
   b. False
   c. True   And has the advantage of treating some of the organisms in non-gonococcal urethritis
   d. False   Serology does not distinguish an acute attack from previous infection
   e. False   This would suggest co-existing syphilis

5. a. False   Although venereal disease is common in the United States, LGV is rare, and usually imported from abroad
   b. True   Although rectal stricture is characteristic
   c. False   The initial penile lesion may escape notice. Later inguinal lymphadenopathy may ulcerate
   d. True
   e. False   It is only slightly penicillin-sensitive

Statistics

1. **In a normal distribution—**
   a. The probability that an observation falls outside 1·96 standard deviations on either side of the mean is 0·01
   b. The mean, mode and median have the same value
   c. Calculation of the variance gives a measure of dispersion
   d. The standard deviation is calculated from the formula
   $$\sqrt{\frac{\Sigma\,(x - \bar{x})}{n-1}}$$
   e. The area under the curve within two standard deviations from the mean is constant, irrespective of the range of the observations

2. **The standard error of the mean—**
   a. Is calculated from the formula
   $$\frac{\text{standard deviation}}{n^2}$$
   b. Is an estimate of the standard deviation that would be obtained from the means of all possible samples of the given size
   c. Is independent of the variation in the population
   d. Is useful in studying the significance of the difference between the means of two samples
   e. Of a sample, drawn from a population which is not normally distributed, is of no value

3. **Correlation—**
   a. Can be illustrated on a scatter diagram
   b. Represented by $r = 1$ implies a perfect positive linear correlation
   c. Represented by $r = 0·5$ implies that 50% of the change in one variable can be accounted for by a change in the other variable
   d. Coefficients can have levels of significance attached which are independent of sample size
   e. Of high degree enables statements about causation to be made

Answers overleaf

1. a. False   The probability of this is 5 per cent or 0·05
    b. True
    c. True   Standard deviation is the square root of the variance
    d. False   If this formula was used negative and positive differences from the mean would cancel out. The correct formula is

$$\sqrt{\frac{\Sigma\,(x - \bar{x})^2}{n-1}}$$

    e. True   It is this fact which enables generalisations about probability to be made

2. a. False   The formula is

$$\frac{\text{standard deviation}}{\sqrt{n}}$$

    b. True
    c. False   The variation of the means of population samples will depend on the variability within the population
    d. True
    e. False   The means of samples drawn from the population may form a normal distribution even where the population does not

3. a. True
    b. True
    c. False r^2 gives an estimate of this, i.e. $(0·5)^2 = 0·25$ or 25%
    d. False   The significance can be estimated by using a t test and to attach a value of probability the degrees of freedom must be known
    e. False   Correlation is not causation

4. **Statistical tests that are non-parametric include—**
   a.   Regression
   b.   Correlation
   c.   The Student's *t* test
   d.   Rank correlation
   e.   Wilcoxon rank sum test

5. **In the *t* test—**
   a.   An estimate of the probability that two samples come from the same population may be obtained
   b.   In estimating the significance of the result the degrees of freedom must be known
   c.   More than 30 observations are required before it can be used
   d.   For a difference to be significant at a given probability, a higher value of *t* is required as the sample size increases
   e.   The distribution of a variable in a sample can be compared with the distribution of that variable in another sample

Answers overleaf

4.   a.   False
      b.   True   Non-parametric tests are ones which can analyse data which are not normally distributed
      c.   False   Non-normally distributed data may be altered (e.g. by logarithms) so as to conform to a normal distribution and enable tests such as the t-test to be used
      d.   True
      e.   True

5.   a.   True
      b.   True
      c.   False   The t-test is adapted for use with small samples
      d.   False
      e.   False   The chi-squared test is used for this

Symptoms and Signs

1. **Causes of palmar erythema include—**
   a. Rheumatoid arthritis
   b. Pregnancy
   c. Hypopituitarism
   d. Multiple sclerosis
   e. Thyrotoxicosis

2. **Extensor plantars and absent ankle jerks are seen in—**
   a. Tabes dorsalis
   b. Friedreich's ataxia
   c. Multiple sclerosis
   d. Parasagittal meningioma
   e. Vitamin B_{12} deficiency

3. **Causes of splinter haemorrhages include—**
   a. Trauma
   b. Hypothyroidism
   c. Trichiniasis
   d. Sarcoidosis
   e. Severe rheumatoid arthritis

4. **Increased skin sweating is a feature of—**
   a. Acromegaly
   b. Cystic fibrosis
   c. Anxiety
   d. Heat stroke
   e. Atropine poisoning

Answers overleaf

1.   a.   True
    b.   True   Excessive oestrogen is also the probable mechanism in liver failure
    c.   False
    d.   False
    e.   True   Chronic febrile illness and chronic leukaemias are the other causes which are quoted

2.   a.   False   Tabes affects the dorsal columns and roots and would cause absent ankle jerks by interrupting the sensory side of the reflex arc. Co-existent general paresis would be required to give the upper motor defect of extensor plantars
    b.   True
    c.   False
    d.   False   This is a cause of spastic paraplegia
    e.   True   A combination of peripheral neuropathy and subacute combined degeneration

3.   a.   True   A much commoner cause than infective endocarditis
    b.   False
    c.   True
    d.   False
    e.   True   They are also found in some skin diseases. Rare causes quoted are malignant neoplasm and mitral stenosis

4.   a.   True
    b.   False   Though the electrolyte content of sweat is abnormal
    c.   True
    d.   False   Loss of the capacity to sweat is one of the problems
    e.   False   Atropine blocks the cholinergic stimulus of normal sweating

5. **Reversed splitting of the second heart sound is a recognised feature of—**
   a. Pulmonary hypertension
   b. Wolff–Parkinson–White syndrome
   c. Aortic stenosis
   d. Left bundle branch block
   e. First degree heart block

6. **Onycholysis is characteristic of—**
   a. Thyrotoxicosis
   b. Psoriasis
   c. Fungal infection of the nails
   d. Syphilis
   e. Nephrotic syndrome

7. **Fine crepitations maximal at the end of inspiration are characteristic of—**
   a. Byssinosis
   b. Bronchiectasis
   c. Pulmonary oedema
   d. Fibrosing alveolitis
   e. α_1-antitrypsin deficiency

8. **Increased melanin pigmentation is a recognised feature of—**
   a. Primary biliary cirrhosis
   b. Chédiak–Higashi syndrome
   c. Haemochromatosis
   d. Renal failure
   e. Hyperthyroidism

Answers overleaf

5. a. False
   b. False The first heart sound may be loud due to the short P–R interval
   c. True   Aortic valve closure is delayed and may follow pulmonary valve closure in expiration. Then in inspiration pulmonary valve closure is delayed and the degree of splitting may narrow
   d. True   Again aortic valve closure is delayed
   e. False The first heart sound is soft

6. a. True   It also occurs in hypothyroidism, though less often
   b. True
   c. True   Trauma is the other common cause. Others are idiopathic
   d. False
   e. False Leuconychia is seen

7. a. False This causes airways obstruction
   b. False Crepitations are coarse
   c. False Crepitations are characteristically early in inspiration in pulmonary oedema
   d. True
   e. False This is associated with emphysema

8. a. True   Melanin pigmentation may be early. Hyperbilirubinaemia may also contribute to skin colour
   b. False Depigmentation is characteristic
   c. True   Iron may also contribute
   d. True   Urochrome also contributes
   e. True   As with other endocrine disorders, e.g. Addison's

9.   **A diastolic murmur of mitral origin may be due to—**
  a.   Atrial septal defect
  b.   Hypertrophic obstructive cardiomyopathy
  c.   Patent ductus arteriosus
  d.   Aortic incompetence
  e.   Pulmonary incompetence

10.   **Recognised causes of Raynaud's phenomenon include—**
  a.   Carcinoid syndrome
  b.   Scleroderma
  c.   Cervical rib
  d.   Cryoglobulinaemia
  e.   Psoriasis

Answers overleaf

9. a. False A tricuspid diastolic murmur may be heard due to increased flow
    b. False The basic murmur is due to aortic outflow obstruction. Mitral incompetence is common later
    c. True   Due to increased flow
    d. True   Probably due to vibration of the anterior cusp by the regurgitant aortic jet (Austin Flint murmur)
    e. False The right-sided equivalent of the Austin Flint is occasionally heard coming from the tricuspid valve

10. a. False Facial flushing is characteristic
    b. True   Other collagen diseases are also associated
    c. True   And other causes of vascular occlusion
    d. True   And other dysproteinaemias
    e. False Do not forget Raynaud's disease, vibrating tools and drugs as other causes